Prevention of Perioperative Infections

Antibiotics and Chemotherapy

Vol. 33

Series Editors
H. Schönfeld, Grenzach
F.E. Hahn, Washington, D.C.

KARGER

S. Karger · Basel · München · Paris · London · New York · Tokyo · Sydney

Prevention of Perioperative Infections

Volume Editor
H. Schönfeld, Grenzach

9 figures and 35 tables, 1985

KARGER

S. Karger · Basel · München · Paris · London · New York · Tokyo · Sydney

Antibiotics and Chemotherapy

National Library of Medicine, Cataloging in Publication
Prevention of perioperative infections
Volume editor, H. Schönfeld. - Basel; New York: Karger, 1985
(Antibiotics and chemotherapy; vol. 33)
Includes index.
1. Antibiotics - therapeutic use 2. Postoperative Complications - prevention and control
3. Premedication 4. Surgical Wound Infection - prevention and control
I. Schönfeld, H. (Hans) II. Series
W1 AN855G v. 33 [WO 185 P944]
ISBN 3-8055-3936-3

Drug Dosage

The authors and the publisher have exerted every effort to ensure that drug selection and dosage set forth in this text are in accord with current recommendations and practice at the time of publication. However, in view of ongoing research, changes in government regulations, and the constant flow of information relating to drug therapy and drug reactions, the reader is urged to check the package insert for each drug for any change in indications and dosage and for added warnings and precautions. This is particularly important when the recommended agent is a new and/or infrequently employed drug.

Printed in Switzerland by Basler Zeitung, Basel
ISBN 3-8055-3936-3

Contents

Foreword

Any book devoted to the prevention of perioperative infections inevitably runs into controversies. Apart from the obvious questions relating to indications, choice of drug, route of administration, timing and duration, the prophylactic use of antibiotics touches such hotly debated issues as hospital costs and their containment, excessive use of medication, real risks versus potential benefits, and the compromises often forced by the fear of malpractice litigation.

That such questions must be answered according to the type of operation involved will be readily apparent in the contributions to this volume, each of which considers the prevention of infections at a particular operative site. Two obvious indications for prophylaxis emerge: those cases where the site of the operation (e.g. surgery of the colon) is associated with a statistically high risk of infection and those other cases where the nature of the surgery (e.g. open heart surgery) means that an infection, however unlikely to occur, could be a fatal complication.

Even in such obvious cases, opinions vary considerably concerning the proper timing and duration of drug administration. The use of prophylactic antibiotics for a week or longer following the operation remains common, a practice which is difficult to justify as either prophylaxis (since the wound is closed by then and thus impermeable to bacteria) or as therapy (since there is no infection to treat).

The introduction of new long-acting antibiotics, such as ceftriaxon, which assure effective concentrations for more than 24 hours following a single application, has brought 'one-shot prophylaxis' back into the foreground of the discussion. As in the past, it remains uncertain which role is played by the anaerobics and whether it is necessary, in particular localizations, to administer anaerobic-effective drugs as an adjuvant measure.

Perhaps most difficult to clarify is the question of knowing when real risks, such as induced resistance and toxic or hypersensitivity reactions, outweigh potential benefits to the patient. Again, the issue is complicated by the pressure of risks to the physician, who may be held responsible should infectious complications arise. The existence of such a risk appears to be one explanation for the practice of administering antibiotics on a preventive basis for up to two weeks following a clearly 'clean' operation.

This volume was put together in an effort to clarify both the beneficial and detrimental effects of measures to prevent infections during or following surgery at different organ sites. Appreciation is expressed to the authors who found the time to communicate their considerable personal experiences in the form of these original contributions. As in past volumes of this series, the editor has refrained from letting his own opinions override the views and experiences of these invited authorities.

Hans Schönfeld

Antibiot. Chemother., vol. 33, pp. 1–29 (Karger, Basel 1985)

Perioperative Prevention of Infection in Genitourinary Surgery

Stacy J. Childs

Community Health Sciences, University of Alabama, Tuscaloosa, Ala., USA; Southeastern Research Foundation, Inc., Birmingham, Ala., USA

Introduction

Urinary tract infections (UTIs) are easily treated. The majority are caused from gram-negative bacteria and respond quite readily to drugs achieving high concentrations in the urine such as sulfa, nitrofurantoin, ampicillin among others. Why then are we so intent on the prevention of infections around the time of urologic surgery if treatment of these simple complications is rather artless? To answer the above question we must peer in depth to the problem.

The incidence and type of infections need to be investigated as well as the morbidity associated with the same. Only then can we accurately identify the etiology of these bacterial invasions and subsquently place emphasis on prevention in particular areas. This chapter will define criteria for placing blame on a surgical procedure as the agent causing infection and infectious complications and seek out controlled studies that will try to pinpoint operations with high incidences of postoperative infections. In addition to categories at risk, we must identify patients with greater likelihood of developing these infections and finally look at treatment. Treatment must be approached from a prevention standpoint indicating procedures, protocols, and anti-infective agents lessening the risks of bacterial invasion. It must then mention appropriate therapeutic regimens once infection or complication has resulted.

The literature contains a multitude of reports for the prevention of urinary tract infections especially associated with the use of indwelling catheters. This chapter shall select those protocols of greater interest and merit upon which to dwell and focus less on the experimental than the practical. The economics of preventing perioperative infections will be dissertated less than probably necessary.

Nosocomial Urinary Tract Infections

Briefly, the problem is this. 3 of every 100 patients that walk into a hospital in the United States will develop an infection that was not present on admission. This 3% nosocomial infection rate has remained virtually the same over the last decade. Approximately 40% of all such infections have their origin in the urinary tract [1]. 70–80% of all of these hospital-born urinary tract infections result from some form of urologic manipulation such as cystocopy, catheterization, or urethral dilatation [2, 3]. It was previously stated that these infections are easily treated with inexpensive drugs and one might dismiss the question entirely were it not for the fact that those patients that acquire a urinary tract infection following such instrumentation have a 3-fold increase in mortality compared to other hospitalized patients [4]. Evidence linking these patients to death rates may in fact be circumstantial; however, let us look at some facts and figures that make the picture more valid.

Approximately 2% of all admissions to our hospitals will develop a urinary tract infection while there. *Escherichia coli* is the most common etiologic organism accounting for close to 50% of the patients with bacteriuria. Other gram negatives such as *Proteus* sp. and *Klebsiella* certainly are present in similar proportions as one sees in community acquired infection. One interesting event has been observed; the longer a patient is in a hospital the smaller percentage these aforementioned bacteria contribute. After being in the hospital for several days, organisms such as *Serratia* and *Pseudomonas* become more common and the percent of *E. coli* and *Proteus* gets smaller [5]. In fact, the entire bacterial population has changed proportions in the last decade or so. We are finding a greater contingent of troublesome organisms such as *Serratia, Pseudomonas, Staphylococcus aureus,* and even enterococcus in the urinary tract and a smaller number of the common community acquired pathogens such as *E. coli* [6].

Table I demonstrates that several organisms causing hospital acquired urinary tract infections are present at rates much different than would be expected in community acquired infections [7]. Group D *Streptococcus, Enterobacter, Serratia* and *Pseudomonas* together ac-

Table I. Rates and relative frequency of selected pathogens causing nosocomial infections, by site of infection, 1978

	Primary bacteremia	Surgical wound	Urinary tract
S. aureus	2.4	15.8	3.2
	(13.8)	(14.6)	(2.0)
S. epidermidis	1.5	4.8	4.9
	(8.9)	(4.4)	(3.1)
S. pneumoniae	0.2	0.1	0.0[1]
	(1.0)	(0.1)	(0.0)[2]
Streptococcus, group A	0.1	0.6	0.1
	(0.7)	(0.6)	(0.0)
Streptococcus, group B	0.5	2.4	2.2
	(2.9)	(2.2)	(1.4)
Streptococcus, group D	1.1	10.4	21.9
	(6.2)	(9.6)	(13.8)
E. coli	2.7	15.7	51.1
	(15.6)	(14.6)	(32.1)
Klebsiella spp.	1.9	5.4	14.5
	(10.9)	(5.0)	(9.1)
Enterobacter spp.	0.9	4.3	6.9
	(5.0)	(3.9)	(4.3)
Proteus-Providencia spp.	0.4	7.5	15.2
	(2.4)	(7.0)	(9.6)
Pseudomonas aeruginosa	1.0	5.7	16.1
	(6.0)	(5.3)	(10.1)
Pseudomonas, other spp.	0.2	1.0	2.6
	(0.9)	(0.9)	(1.6)
Serratia spp.	0.5	1.3	4.1
	(3.1)	(1.2)	(2.6)
Bacteroides fragilis	0.6	3.9	0.0[1]
	(3.5)	(3.6)	(0.0)[2]
Secondary bacteremia	NA	4.2	4.5
	(-)[2]	(3.9)	(2.8)

Rate is number of isolates reported per 10,000 patients discharged; up to 4 isolates may be reported per infection.
Relative frequency is expressed as percent of all isolates from each site.
[1] Incidence is less than 0.1 per 10,000 discharge.
[2] Relative frequency is less than 0.1% of all isolates from that site.

count for as many infections as does *E. coli* in a hospital setting. The changing scope of hospital bacteria may be due to several reasons, despite better technique in catheterization and technological improvements in facilities. The use, misuse, or over-use of antimicrobials and newer powerful anti-infective agents probably has changed the virulence of these organisms to a great degree.

The fact that we have a large number of nosocomial urinary tract infections caused from a changing group of organisms usually related to urologic instrumentation would not be of great importance were it not for the following alarming and irrefutable points. Although the rate of primary bacteremia admissions to the hospitals has remained virtually unchanged throughout the decade of the 1970s in the United States, the rate of secondary bacteremia, i.e. bacteremia resulting from a separate primary source of infection such as the urinary tract, has tripled [1]! About 1% of patients with hospital-born urinary tract infections will experience bacteremia while in the hospital and 10% of those will die [2]. Considering the entire problem of gram-negative bacteremia, approximately 75% is hospital acquired and related to urologic instrumentation, vascular catheters or mechanical ventilation [8]. The frequency of gram-negative bacteremia has increased dramatically in many institutions over the last 20 or 30 years and now must be considered one of the most frequent types of lethal infections in the United States. In a urologic practice this is by far the commonest type of serious life-threatening infection observed [8, 9]!

The topic has become an important one. Infections of the genitourinary tract consistently rank among the top 10 discharge diagnoses in community and university hospitals alike. Were these infections community acquired or outside of the hospital setting there would surely be lack of concern. But, because the urinary tract is implicated in such a high percentage of hospital-born infections and the organisms and sites involved have been repeatedly incriminated as causative for the increase in secondary bacteremia and increasing mortality, we must now address the principal contributor to the matter.

Urologic Instrumentation and Catheterization

Obsolete open catheter drainage invariably led to bacteriuria in a majority of patients within 2 or 3 days. The most obvious source was the drainage receptacle. Even with the advent of newer closed drainage systems, the rate of bacteriuria has continued to increase at the rate of 5–10% each day that a Foley catheter remains indwelling; the end point being that virtually all patients with indwelling Foley catheters will eventually be infected [10–12]. Other forms of urologic instrumentation such as urethral dilatation, cystoscopy and transurethral surgery can result in bacteriuria in from 10 to 50% of the time [13–15].

These unacceptably high rates of bacteriuria following manipulation of the urinary tract become more important when realizing how common urethral procedures and catherization are today. 5–16% of patients in community hospitals have Foley catheters [3, 10–12]. In fact, it is currently estimated that almost a million nosocomial urinary tract infections occur annually as a result of such instrumentation and catheterization in the United States among the total of 40 million patients hospitalized. Those who acquire a hospital-born urinary tract infection can expect increased morbidity with longer hospital stays, and increased costs in the thousands of dollars [2, 16, 17]. Although many cases of catheter or instrument associated bacteriuria are asymptomatic, at least 1–2% will be associated with secondary bacteremia and the fatality rate for nosocomial urinary tract infections is 1% [2, 14] (table II)!

Although most of these infections may be asymptomatic and seemingly require little skill to treat, they contribute an enormous burden to the health care system. Without regard to the added costs of bacteremia such as intensive care services, intravenous fluids, drugs for treating shock and excluding physicians' fees and extra laboratory tests, these

Table II. Incidence, morbidity, and mortality of nosocomial UTIs

40 million admissions to US hospitals yearly
1 million develop nosocomial UTIs
75–80% result from urologic catheterization or instrumentation
5–16% of patients in community hospitals are catheterized
Bacteriuria increases 5–10% per day of catheterization
Cystoscopy or urologic instrumentation produces a 10–50% infection rate
Secondary bacteremia has tripled in 1970s
75% of patients with gram-negative bacteremia related to urologic instrumentation, catheters or ventilators
1% of nosocomial UTIs develop bacteremia and 10% of these will die

simple nosocomial UTIs may add over $31.00 per occupied bed per month [18]. Thus, a 500-bed hospital, 80% occupied, could expect additional overhead of approximately $150,000.00 a year for these trivial infections!

What organisms should we expect to cause these instrument-associated UTIs? *E. coli* is certainly the most common nosocomial urinary pathogen but at a frequency of less than 50% that seen in an outpatient environment. *Serratia, Pseudomonas, Providentia, Morganella, Citrobacter* and enterococcus are much more important in the hospitalized-instrumented patient and become especially effectual in the incontinent bed-ridden patient who has received antibiotics [19, 20]. *Fowler* [3] has postulated that catheter associated UTIs are derived from urethral flora because of increased bacterial colonization of the urethra.

The normal bowel flora contain many bacteria that may be pathogenic in the urinary tract. These colonic organisms, as well as those acquired during hospitalization, have been associated with subsequent UTIs in catheterized patients [21-24]. A variety of gram-negative and gram-positive bacteria normally colonize the distal urethra and periurethral mucosa of female adults, but the male urethra is usually colonized by gram-positive bacteria [25]. The prostate may harbor potentially pathogenic bacteria, however, and approximately 5% of males carry enterobacteriaceae in the urethra. Isolation of *E. coli* from males with urethral catheters undergoing prostatectomy is more common postoperative than preoperative [27]. Not surprisingly, gram-negative bacilli or enterococcus has been isolated from the meatus in as much as 30% of catheterized males. Urethral or meatal colonization is extremely important and preceeds bacteriuria in catheterized-instrumented patients. The density, however, is more suasive in predicting bacteriuria than mere prevalence [29].

The infecting organisms probably originate from the patient's own bacterial flora but may be transmitted between catheterized patients by passive carriage on the hands of noncolonized hospital personnel [30]. Bacteria which do not often colonize the colon would be examples [31, 32]. Cross-examination of urinary catheters has more than once been incriminated in nosocomial outbreaks of *Serratia* and *Proteus* [30, 33-35]. Even more disturbing is the report of 38 cases of multidrug-resistant *Serratia marcescens* largely restricted to patients on a urology service. Although 3 of the patients had indwelling bladder catheters and developed their infection apparently from cross-contamination the majority developed their infection through urologic instrumentation. Contamination of the cystoscope disinfectant solution was eventually discovered. Most of the patients were symptomatic and 2 in fact were bacteremic [36].

Knowing the dominant pathogens and their likely provenance, we must examine the portals of entry. Aside from subsistent prostatic or urethral bacteria, other sources of gram-positive contamination associated with genitourinary surgery can be predicted. The cystoscopy room itself can potentially serve as a reservoir of gram-positive or gram-negative growth [14]. As expected, passage of a single urethral catheter (or instrument) in females has been shown in some studies to be associated with the development of infection [37–39]. There is presumptive evidence that the rate of infection may be greater in a hospital setting than an outpatient ambulatory population [40].

Possible entry points for bacteria in a closed drainage system include the urethral meatus, the catheter-drainage tube junction and the drainage bag itself [4]. The latter can become contaminated as a consequence of inadequate aseptic insertion, contaminated instruments, periurethral colonization, junctional disconnection or irrigation as well as transient organisms in the urine which multiply within the bag [42]. Although catheter reservoir bacterial growth has been proven to play a role [23, 33], bladder infections arising from the same may have been over-estimated [43–45]. On the other hand, contamination at the catheter-drainage tube junction is frequent [10, 11, 46].

Easily the largest contribution to catheter-associated nosocomial urinary tract infections lies at the catheter-urethral junction for the reasons indicated previously [3, 29, 42]. However, contamination from urologic instrumentation with or without an associated catheter also influences bacteriuria and bacteremia. We will explore studies on the efficacy of antibiotic prophylaxis for urologic surgery later in this chapter but a few points are needed at this time. First, only in the last decade, particularly in the past 5 years, have there been well-designed controlled clinical trials to test and illustrate true infection rates from genitourinary surgery. Second it is important to emphasize that short term prophylactic antibiotics or meticulous sterile techniques have little to do with the long range incidence of bacteriuria [47].

If one uses day 5 as the final evaluation point for correlating procedure and antibiotic with the infection rate, the long-debated question is finally resolved. Patients undergoing urologic surgical procedures receiving placebo (no antibiotics) preoperatively and/or perioperatively develop postoperative bacteriuria from 20 to 37% of the time in the most conservative of calculations. There are statistically significant differences between placebo and antibiotic groups and we shall discuss this further below. An equally important consideration is that in at least one study involving open prostatectomy there was a 12% wound infection rate among the nonantibiotic patients. The major threat and concern of course, is the discovery that postoperative bacteremia is as high as 25% among placebo patients. Sepsis is from 1 to 8% in five different studies among nonantibiotic patients undergoing urologic instrumentation [13, 17, 48–53]. Several of these investigations show significantly increased costs and days of hospitalization as a result of these infections and infectious complications.

At Greater Risk of Infection

There are certain situational and individual characteristics that categorize the patient into higher than normal risks (table III, IV). Many of these have been mentioned elsewhere and most can be known preoperatively so that infection in the perioperative period is anticipated. Situational influences include the presence of an indwelling catheter or being placed in a room, ward or unit with infected patients – particularly catheterized patients with UTIs [30].

Table III. Situations that place patients at increased risk for infection

Indwelling catheter
Infected roomate (especially catheterized)
Preoperative shaving
Prolonged preoperative hospitalization
Surgery
Poor technique
Contaminated equipment
Prolonged operation
Increased blood loss
Improper drainage
Excessive cautery
Necrotic debris

Even the preoperative shaving of the operative field may prejudice toward infection [54]. Surgery itself can inhibit systemic host defenses - neutrophil and lymphocyte function - and a long preoperative stay may adversely bias the outcome. Other situations in which the patient may have little control include the use of contaminated equipment or prosthesis, skill of the surgeon, the duration and blood loss of the surgery and anesthesia influences. The improper use of drains or inadequately sized urethral catheters can affect drainage of fluid or blood (hematomas) giving way to environments favoring bacterial growth. Over-use of the electrocautery in open or transurethral procedures or leaving behind necrotic debris such as prostate 'chips' also may result in a situation favoring infection. Obviously, the patient can neither govern the amount of normal nor nonviable tissue inoculated.

Often overlooked by urologists, author included, is the surgical mask and proper surgical scrub prior to transurethral procedures. The potential of contaminating the exterior of sterile gloves exists anytime self-gloving occurs, not to mention the possibility of manufacturing flaws in the material [58]. A mask should probably be worn as a barrier between the face and resectoscope if it is important between face and scalpel [59]. Tape, manufactured on the mask or applied, can keep the lens from fogging.

The individual traits that place the patient at greater risks of infection are more numerous and complex. In general, a history of recurrent urinary tract infections or prostatitis, pregnancy, female sex and in-

Table IV. Individual characteristics placing patients at greater risk of infection

History of recurrent UTIs or prostatitis
Pregnancy
Female
Elderly
Serious underlying disease or disability
Malnutrition
Hematologic disorders
Poorly controlled diabetes
Rheumatoid arthritis
Co-existing infection
Cancer

creasing age all are associated with greater chance of infection in a surgical setting. The occurrence of bacterial UTI increases approximately 1% per decade of age. Patients with underlying diseases, the chronically ill or debilitated and the malnourished likewise are jeopardized [4, 19, 55]. 1 out of 3 hospitalized adults suffers from protein-calorie malnutrition. These patients have greater susceptibility to infection and the resultant mortality from sepsis is increased. Such patients may have defects in complement system, polymorphonuclear leukocyte (PMN) function and serum/secretory antibody responses [60].

The whole concept of the prevention of perioperative infections was explained by *Miles* [61], *Evans* et al. [62] and *Miles* et al. [63] almost 3 decades ago when 'host resistance' was exhalted and its inhibition gained distinction as the enhancement of bacterial lesions. They showed that interruption of the complement system or ischemia at an operative site did not precede and cause infection. Rather, the interruption occurred immediately after bacterial contamination and the dilemma was repaired promptly when the physiology of the area normalized.

Contemporary studies have shown that the anergic patient undergoing major surgery runs a 1 in 3 chance of major sepsis unless correction of suppressed host defense mechanisms is accomplished. The hosts' defenses are made up of an antibody component (B lymphocytes), a cell-mediated component (T lymphocytes), a phagocytic component (PMNs, macrophages, reticuloendothelial system) and complement. Derangements or inadequacies in these defenses can be blamed for a variety of conditions that should be a red flag to surgeons. Poorly controlled diabetics, patients with rheumatoid arthritis or those with co-existing bacterial or viral infections are at greater risks for infection [60, 64]. Also at danger are patients receiving steroids, anticancer or immunosuppressive drugs and patients with virtually any hematologic disorder. Individuals with cancer, especially lymphoreticular neoplasms, are in potentially perilous positions if undergoing surgery [65, 66].

Prevention of Infection

Having gone over the pathogenesis of perioperative urinary tract infections and concluding that this is a highly significant problem both from the morbidity and from an economic standpoint, it is now advisable to go into specific areas where physicians can make a favorable impact. The area of genitourinary surgical antibiotic prophylaxis will be discussed in considerable depth later in this chapter. From the preceeding data, however, it becomes quite obvious that as the catheter and urologic instruments seem to play a major role in the development of these infections, the first and perhaps major theme should be 'do not catheterize nor urologically instrument unless absolutely necessary'. Realizing that cystoscopy or urethral dilatation as a diagnostic tool or treatment carries certain risks and expenses, urologists should carefully weigh these procedures in the balance of cost-complication versus benefit. Equally, urethral catheters should not be inserted merely for the ease or convenience of patients, nursing personnel or physicians. The catheter should be used when absolutely necessary and careful individual consideration should be given to each case. If a catheter is then elected, one with a diameter as narrow as possible should be inserted to allow secretions to drain more freely [67]. Alternatives such as intermittent catheterization or a shorter interval of catheterization should be considered [5, 68].

A host of data can be found in the urologic literature on the potential for prevention of catheter-associated infections. We have reviewed this quite exhaustively and have found similar conclusions as others [5, 41, 69]. The recommendations that follow include measures that are strongly supported by well-designed and controlled clinical studies as well as those that are supported by highly suggestive clinical studies. A certain amount of practicality must be employed when looking at these guidelines such that we do not allow the costs of prevention to far outweigh the costs of treatment. There may be some slight variances that will be included from the author based on such practicality and extensive personal experience in county as well as community hospitals.

The Centers for Disease Control has summarized their recommendations for catheter care in 12 categories. These along with my further suggestions are listed below [69]:

Personnel

Only persons (hospital personnel, family members or patients) who are familiar with and have been thoroughly checked out in the procedure of aseptic catheterization and maintenance should handle catheters. These persons should be given periodic in-service training and be aprised of the complications associated with urinary catheterization.

Catheter Use

The smallest diameter catheter should be used as is practical for the purpose or procedure involving catheterization. Catheters should be used only when absolutely necessary and not merely as a convenience for the patient, personnel, or physician. A catheter should be left indwelling as short a period of time as possible and alternative methods of urinary drainage should be considered. Suprapubic catheterization or intermittent urethral catheterization can be satisfactory alternatives to the indwelling catheter and in some cases condom catheter drainage may be preferred. Unless strict meticulous condom catheter care is employed, however, it is our experience that the infection rate is not only as great but that skin problems or phimosis may become significant complications.

Hand Washing

Hand washing is recommended immediately before and after catheterization or any manipulation of the catheter, the meatus, or catheter-drainage receptacle apparatus. When personnel are manipulating as above it is advisable that gloves be used (clean but not necessarily sterile) and that they be discarded before leaving the room.

Catheter Insertion

Only sterile catheters should be inserted and the technique aseptic. All supplies including gloves, drape, sponges and antiseptic periurethral cleansing solutions as well a lubricant jelly should be single use varieties. A catheter should be secured under little or no tension to prevent movement and urethral traction.

Drainage

Only sterile, continuously closed drainage systems should be used and the system should not be disconnected unless the catheter must be irrigated. Sterile technique should be employed whenever the system is opened for irrigation. If breaks in aseptic technique, disconnection, or leakage occur any contaminated systems should be immediately replaced with new sterile systems.

Irrigation

Irrigation should be avoided unless obstruction is anticipated such as following transurethral prostate or bladder surgery. Closed continuous irrigation can be used to prevent obstruction. An intermittent method may be used to remove clots or other obstructions but attention to sterile technique in changing irrigation fluid is essential. Although reports in the literature list for and against conclusions about continuous irrigation with antimicrobials, recent opinion is that this is not necessary and may even foster the development of resistant bacteria.

Specimen Collection

Small volumes of urine for culture can be aspirated from the distal catheter using a sterile syringe and small gauge needle or obtained from the sample port of the drainage tubing. The area should be cleansed with disinfectant beforehand. Large volumes of urine for special chemical analysis should be obtained aseptically from the drainage bag.

Urinary Flow

Unobstructed 'downhill' flow must be maintained at all times. The catheter must be kept from kinking and the collecting bag must be emptied regularly. The collecting bag must always be kept below the level of the bladder. Catheter change is necessary when concretions can be detected or flow becomes obstructed.

Meatal Care

Once or twice daily perineal care includes cleansing of the meatal catheter junction with an antiseptic soap solution. An antimicrobial ointment may be applied but the efficacy for preventing infection has not been proven. This may serve more as a lubricant to decrease trauma.

Catheter Change Interval

Chronic indwelling catheters need to be changed only when concretions develop or the catheter becomes obstructed or malfunctions. Symptomatic infections, when treated, should have catheter change accompanying the antibiotics.

Spacial Separation of Catheterized Patients

Catheterized patients should be separated from each other whenever possible and especially if one is bacteriuric.

Bacteriologic Monitoring

Daily bacteriologic monitoring is probably not necessary. Patients usually asymptomatic such as nursing home patients with chronic indwelling catheters should certainly have bacterial cultures performed if they become symptomatic or febrile. Postoperative patients with catheters indwelling should havc bacterial cultures performed every 2 days while catheter is in place for the first 5 or 6 days. After that time period infection is likely. The catheter should be removed if possible and single dose therapy given or the patient should then be treated while the catheter is indwelling until it can be removed. Patients should not be treated for prolonged periods! This regimen only applies to postoperative patients, however, and the preceding statements about catheterized nonsurgical patients should be adhered to. Cultures should be performed when the catheter is removed if feasible.

Several authors have shown that colony counts as low as 10^3 CFU/ml in the postoperative patient require attention as do mixed infections. Many of these do not clear without treatment and several become 'silently septic' with serious morbidity.

Instillation of substances such as hydrogen peroxide, povodine iodine, neomycin among others should not be placed into the drainage bags as reports on decreasing bacteriuria have been refuted. Nonoperative patients with indwelling catheters who are in high risks categories are certainly candidates for more frequent bacteriologic monitoring.

Although the above recommendations are important for the prevention of these infections, when bacteriuria occurs it is essential that a few principles be followed. First, asymptomatic bacteriuria in a chronic indwelling catheter does not necessarily require antibiotics except in high risks persons. Single or multiple dose antibiotics at the time the catheter is removed is probably adequate for the treatment of bacteriuria in patients catheterized for short periods of time. Catheterized postoperative patients who develop bacteriuria, symptomatic or not, should either have their catheters immediately removed and repeat cultures performed with very close monitoring of the patient or they should be treated with appropriate antimicrobials.

Genitourinary Surgical Prophylaxis

Genitourinary surgical prophylaxis is the use of antimicrobials to reduce the risk of infectious complications. Its goal, therefore, is not only to decrease the short-term incidence of postoperative bacteriuria but, hopefully, to show less incidence of sepsis and wound infection. Of paramount importance is that physicians do no harm with their method of prophylaxis. That is, by administering a drug, authorizing a catheter protocol or employing an infection control regimen such as the movement or isolation of a patient, we must strive to complete a patient's stay in the hospital without damage.

Patient damage can be a drug reaction or side effect. Nephrotoxicity, bleeding abnormalities, rash and itching, diarrhea or anaphylaxis certainly are undesired. Financial damage may result from the treatment or correction of adverse reactions, from the use of unnecessary drugs, equipment or procedures as well as the withholding of those that are needed.

Equally important is the necessity to assure that the number and type of nosocomial infections are not altered adversely. Surely, significant financial and morbid consequences would ensue if damage to the hospital environment occurred from the over-use or misuse of prophylaxis measures.

Selecting Antimicrobials

In evaluating drugs for use in prophylaxis, the first requirement is safety [71]. Agents associated with a significant incidence of toxicity or side effect should be discouraged. Even though these untoward reactions may usually be seen after multiple days or doses, the stress, blood loss or anesthesia of surgery should make surgeons anticipate the unexpected responses. If a drug chosen for prophylaxis has a 20% chance of a significant side effect and the surgical procedure carrys a 10% risk of minor infection, one might opt for the gamble of postoperative therapy rather than prevention.

Next, the drug selected must be appropriate for the operative site [71]. When choosing a prophylactic agent for major bowel surgery such as ileal or sigmoid conduit diversion, an antibiotic covering the intestinal flora is preferred over one covering the bacteria of the urethra or prostate. Transurethral surgery on the other hand concerns itself with community and hospital gram-negatives and in certain cases, *S. aureus, Staphylococcus saprophyticus* and *Streptococcus faecalis*.

A frequently made error is to select an agent that only achieves bactericidal urine levels for urologic prophylaxis [72–76]. Although urine concentration is helpful and important, bactericidal levels of the drug also should be attained in the serum as well as the tissue operated upon [15]. Bactericidal concentration in these 3 areas and appropriate bacterial spectrum of the drug used must be a desired prerequisite for urologic prophylaxis.

The timing of an antibiotic is critical. Experimental studies from the 1950s hold true today. Maximum effectiveness in preventing surgical infections is achieved only when the drug has been given before surgery. Adequate urine, serum and tissue levels are needed at incision time as well as throughout surgery [63, 77].

The National Research Council has created a classification of wounds with corresponding infection rates [78, 79]. The following definitions and expanded genitourinary applications help us decide precisely when to use antibiotic prophylaxis (table V). One must remember that high risk patients or patients receiving any prosthetic device such as penile or testicular prosthesis or graft material, are candidates for antibiotic prophylaxis because of the financial and morbid consequences should infection occur.

Clean Operations

These are procedures where there is no unusual contamination nor crossing of a mucous membrane. The infection rate is considered less than 5%. There is ordinarily no entry to the urinary tract and this includes procedures such as orchiectomy, varicocele repair (or internal spermatic vein ligation) and cystourethropexy without entering the urinary tract. No antibiotic prophylaxis is indicated in this category.

Clean-Contaminated Operations

These imply crossing of mucosae (entry to the urinary tract) and can be associated with an infection rate as high as 10%. Prophylaxis would not normally be indicated here except in the high risk situations previously mentioned. Procedures include nephrectomy, ureterolithotomy, cystectomy or cystotomy among others. I hasten to point out that patients in any category with known or suspected bacteriuria, regardless of the colony count, would demand therapy, not prophylaxis!

Contaminated Operations

These cases are associated with acute, nonpurulent inflammation or a break in sterile technique. The infection rate is 20% or more and must include all transurethral surgery where the mucosae of the uri-

Table V. Recommendations for antibiotic prophylaxis in genitourinary surgery [14]

Operative wound classification	Infection risk, %	Recommendations
Clean Orchiectomy Anterior cystourethropexy Varicocelectomy	< 5	no prophylaxis (exceptions: prosthesis or foreign body insertion, cystourethropexy involving cystoscopy or vaginal manipulation)
Clean-contaminated Ureterolithotomy Pyelolithotomy Nephrectomy Partial cystectomy Cystotomy	10	prophylaxis only in high-risk patients (elderly, malnourished, debilitated, diabetic, immunosuppressed, patients with prosthetic devices)
Contaminated TURP and other invasive transurethal procedures (sterile urine preoperatively) Ileal or sigmoid conduit with proper bowel preparation	20	prophylaxis (exception: cystoscopy, simple retrograde pyelography)
Dirty Any procedure following acute trauma TURP or other urethral procedures in the presence of bacteriuria Ileocystoplasty, ureterosigmoidostomy or ileal conduit in absence of adequate bowel preparation	at least 30	prophylaxis followed by postoperative treatment regimen

nary tract is invaded. The procedure being performed in a 'dirty' cystoscopy room along with the inevitable lens-eye contact multiply the inherent risks of abrasion of an infected or colonized prostate and/or urethra. Operations here would also include 'properly prepared' bowel cases such as conduit diversion or augmentation cystoplasty as well as percutaneous endoscopy. Prophylaxis is advisable in this category. Exceptions might be occasionally found in young, healthy individuals receiving brief stay or outpatient surgery.

Dirty Operations

Here we include acute trauma or transurethral procedures in the presence of infection. Bowel surgery in the absence of satisfactory preparation would fall into this category. The infection rate may be 30% or more and since it is expected, therapy – not prophylaxis alone – is indicated. Antibiotics should be given both preoperatively and in a postoperative therapeutic regimen when possible.

Once more, an important point must be understood and implemented in addition to all of the preceding principals in this chapter. The presence or detection of any bacteria in an operative site, regardless of the colony count, dictates placing a patient in a therapeutic category from a prophylactic one. Readers may have experienced the following scenario which has occurred in my practice several times over the years. A patient is admitted for elective transurethral prostatic surgery the day before his operation. That evening, urine is collected for culture but the report is not received before the operation has been completed and a prophylactic regimen implemented. The night or day following surgery the patient becomes restless or confused, febrile or otherwise showing early signs of bacteremia. The preoperative urine culture now is reported as 10,000 colonies of a gram-negative rod. Patients such as this will often be prophylactic 'failures' and must be treated as if an open wound were inoculated with the pathogen. Several days of a therapeutic regimen of the selected antimicrobial which achieves appropriate serum and tissue levels should be given.

We have successfully tried 2 methods to assure that patients are abacteriuric prior to surgery. In smaller hospitals, cultures can be checked by the bacteriologist before scheduled surgery commences and all positive cultures, regardless of colony count, called to the operating room. The urologist or his staff can call the laboratory or operating room throughout the day to check these results which may initiate a therapy regimen.

A preferred method involves having a culture performed in the urologists's office or hospital laboratory within 48 h of surgery and making sure that the result is known within the immediate perioperative period (2 or 3 h). Remember that technical mistakes can be made in reading cultures, transferring the results to a bacteriology report form or delivery of the latter to the chart. Good clinical assessment of the patient preoperatively and judgement of the situation postoperatively can be life-saving.

One recent example comes to mind; an elderly male was admitted to the hospital complaining of marked prostatism. He had been in a small community hospital 6 weeks previously in urinary retention and acquired a nosocomial pseudomonas urinary tract infection at that time. The infection was eradicated with appropriate antibiotics. Upon this admission the patient's urinalysis was negative and his urine culture was reported as 'no growth at 24 h'. Cystoscopy the day after admission revealed obstruction of the prostate and a transurethral resection was performed the following day. The final urine culture 48 h after collection, which was received the afternoon of the patient's surgery, revealed *Pseudomonas* of a colony count of $> 10^5$. The patient was septic within 6 h postoperatively despite receiving adequate antibiotic prophylaxis.

A thorough discussion with the bacteriologist involved in the case revealed that the positive culture had been noted within the first 24 h on the log book and no explanation could be found nor was offered for the negative report on the chart! The point here is that given the patient's history of *Pseudomonas* infection in the situation of prostatic obstruction, this patient was probably doomed to fail prophylaxis. Antibiotics probably should have been started 24 h before surgery and continued for several days postoperatively and should have been based on the culture report of 6 weeks earlier *(Pseudomonas)*. First signs of bacteremia or sepsis should initiate prompt and thorough therapeutic antibiotic methods regardless of culture data. Patients with recent infection, high suspicion for infection or who in fact have positive cultures should all be excluded from prophylaxis. Antibiotic prophylaxis in genitourinary surgery implys achieving adequate urine, tissue, and serum levels of antimicrobials to eradicate small numbers of microbes inoculated at the time of surgery or which may be present in the operative site in numbers undetectable by normal laboratory bacteriologic methods.

Examining the literature and one's own urologic practice makes it obvious that patients with chronic bacteriuria or with a long indwelling preoperative catheter have a higher postoperative infection and sepsis rate [47]. It should now be understood that the preoperative culture must be 'negative' for any bacteria to qualify a patient for prophylaxis over therapeutics. But what is a negative urine culture? Just as the magic 100,000 number indicating significant bacteriuria is meaningless for symptomatic patients, a report of 'no growth' or 'negative' may be meaningless in surgical patients. Some hospitals call $< 10^5$ as negative. It is not unusal for $\leqq 10^4$ to not only be called 'no growth' but for sensitivities to be lacking – a disasterous problem when your patient is septic and the only information you have is '8,000 colonies of a gram-negative rod'! In fact, is the significant level of bacteriuria below that detectable by ordinarily available bacteriology laboratories? We are presently engaged in studies to answer this question.

The problem of which drugs to use, when to start them and how long to continue them is better known now than ever before. *Chodak and Plaut* [80], in their excellent review of the urologic prophylactic literature, have discounted the usefulness of the earlier studies evaluating urologic antibiotic prophylaxis mostly because of poor study design. Inappropriate drugs were often compared in uncontrolled studies for variable dosing schedules involving different surgical procedures. The classic article directed the need for better investigations. The last 5 years have seen the appearance of attempts at improving study design. The first was a double-blind, prospective, placebo-controlled study utilizing cefoxitin perioperatively and as long as a catheter was indwelling postoperatively. Omitting long range incidence of bacteriuria, 26% of placebo patients were infected within 3 postoperative days compared to 4% in the cefoxitin group. Editoral comment by *Kunin* emphasized an extremely important fact; that extended use of an antibiotic may lead to infection from pathogens resistant to the drug [13].

At least 6 other international studies deserve attention. *Prokocimer* et al. [48] showed short-term infection rates of 35 and 3% respectively, for placebo and cefotaxime with a 25% bacteremia rate (1% septic shock) in the former. *Korbel and Maher* [49] demonstrated a 37% infection rate among placebo patients receiving urethral instrumentation whereas only 5% receiving antibiotics became infected. *Shah* et al. [50] showed short-term placebo infection rates of 28% compared to 1% each for 3 oral antibiotics. 4% of placebos were judged septic. The studies of *Goldwasser* et al. [52, 53] resulted in placebo infection rates of 32 and 19.4% for transurethral prostatic surgery and transurethral bladder surgery, respectively, and an 8% incidence of sepsis for the former. Antibiotic groups, again, were spared this unacceptable incidence. Our own studies with placebo controls in transurethral surgery have revealed at least 19% placebo infection rates compared to 2–7% antibiotic group infection rates. No candidates acceptable for antibiotic prophylaxis have become septic compared to a 2% sepsis rate among all

Table VI. Postoperative infection rates in studies of perioperative prophylaxis [14]

Drug	Prophylactic regimen	Type of surgery	Infection rate	
			% infected	number of patients
Placebo	saline preoperative only	TU (male)	19	21
vs.		TU and open	30	49
ceftriaxone	1 g preoperative only	TU (male)	0	26
		TU and open	5	43
Placebo	saline pre- and perioperative	TU	28.9	45
vs.				
aztreonam	1 g pre- and perioperative	TU	6	50
Cefotaxime	regimen 1: 1 g pre- and perioperative	TU and open	13.3	45
vs.	regimen 2: 1 g preoperative + 24 h	TU and open	11.1	45
cefazolin	1 g preoperative + 24 h	TU and open	20.9	43
Cefotaxime	1 g preoperative	TU and open	12.5	48
vs.				
cefoxitin	2 g preoperative + 24 h	TU and open	21.3	47
Cefotaxime	1 g pre- and perioperative	TU and open	3.9	51
vs.				
mezlocillin	4 g pre- and perioperative	TU and open	6.8	44
Cefotaxime	1 g pre- and perioperative	TU and open	11	81
vs.				
piperacillin	2 g pre- and perioperative	TU and open	9	80
Cefotaxime	1 g pre- and perioperative	TU	0	45
vs.				
ceftazidime	1 g preoperative only	TU	2.2	45

Preoperative = 30–90 min before surgery; perioperative = 1–3 doses within first 12 h; postoperative + 24 h = dosing every 6–8 h postoperative for 24 h.,

Table VII. Antibiotic susceptibility – urine isolates

Organisms	Number of isolates	% of species	% of urines	Cumulative, %	Amik	Ampi
E. coli	22,076	67	40	40	98	70
P. aeruginosa	4,969	35	9	49	87	1
Enterococcus	4,441	49	8	57	–	95
Klebsiella pneumoniae	4,214	44	8	65	98	5
Proteus mirabilis	4,222	45	8	73	97	87
S. epidermidis	2,872	21	5	78	–	34
Enterobacter sp.	1,643	26	3	81	99	10
S. aureus	935	5	2	83	–	18
S. marcescens	594	24	1	84	–	5

Data from 150 hospitals throughout the continental US during the period June, July and August 1984. Susceptibility not shown when fewer than 350 isolates were tested. Reprinted with permission of BAC-DATA Medical Information Systems, Inc., Totowa, N.J.

placebo patients [17, 51]. Although sepsis rates are low (usually 2% or less), mortality can be significant if antibiotic cover is not provided [81] (table VI).

Four highly pertinent facts have arisen from our extensive investigation of cephalosporins (first, second, third generation), fourth generation penicillins and monobactams for prophylaxis. First, antibiotics with not only broad spectra but those covering nosocomial pathogens are theoretically preferred but even older drugs such as cefazolin are superior to placebos [17, 82, 83]. Omitting nosocomial or more resistant pathogens from antibiotic cover may be dangerous and borders on walking a medicolegal tightrope (see table VII for example of antibiotic susceptibility). Second, strictly gram-negative drugs are effective most of the time but would be ill-advised in a hospital where enterococcus is a problem or where cephalosporins are abused [51]. Next, enterococcal coverage seems to be advised in elderly patients from nursing homes or other convalescent facilities who have indwelling catheters [20]. And, finally, there does not appear to be any difference in efficacy between perioperative dosing schedules and a single dose preoperative regimen of these powerful antibiotics [17, 84]. Resistance to these anti-

Carb	Cfox	Cfop	Cman	Ctax	Gent	Moxl	Mzlo	Ntro	Pipr	Tmsz	Torb
75	96	95	94	98	98	99	83	96	84	93	98
72	2	78	1	22	78	42	68	1	91	9	88
89	3	–	11	–	44	–	–	93	98	72	41
7	94	–	91	99	95	98	–	60	79	89	95
93	97	–	96	97	97	99	–	14	95	94	97
–	76	–	91	–	80	–	–	95	–	71	79
71	9	–	57	–	95	–	–	56	–	90	95
–	–	–	–	–	89	–	–	–	–	92	–
51	–	–	–	–	64	–	–	7	–	68	57

microbials has not been copious when used in this manner and would not be expected. On the contrary, resistance to an antibiotic can be assured in a setting where multiple, repeated exposure of a pathogen to the drug occurs [85]. Potent and less widely used drugs for therapeutics seem to offer the most promise for prophylaxis. Frequently used antibiotics for therapy but less effective for nosocomial pathogens are definitely the poorer choice for antibiotic prophylaxis in genitourinary surgery.

Presently, two-thirds of urologists utilize some form of genitourinary surgical antibiotic prophylaxis although many do so inappropriately [86, 87]. Precise surveillance and monitoring may lessen infection rates in patients without benefit of prophylaxis but this is certainly the exception rather than the rule. A few reports discourage the use of antibiotic prophylaxis but these share common flaws [76, 85, 88]. First, they do not include analysis of the current literature and/or their conclusions have been based upon poorly designed studies. The doctrine of advising prophylaxis only for patients with positive urine cultures is to recommend seat belts only for drivers who have automobile accidents. That's therapy not prophylaxis. It is also denying significance to a 1–8% sepsis rate and a 20–40% infection rate – clearly unacceptable in a community urologic practice. The costs of single dose or even perioperative schedules of antibiotics are far less than those associated with the consequences of withholding prophylaxis. Patients developing simple postoperative infections may incur minimum costs of treatment but those with serious infections or sepsis may have liabilities in the thousands of dollars [17, 48, 52, 81].

Discussions on the merits of various drugs can be found elsewhere [14] (table VI) but a few points are advisable here. Probably thousands of patients would need to be entered in double-blinded trials to show statistically significant differences among many commonly used antibiotics. Practical guidelines of effectiveness and safety should be employed to select a protocol (elaborated earlier). Try to avoid potentially toxic compounds or those with adverse reactions complicating a surgical course. Nephrotoxic drugs may be more so during the hypotension of anesthesia or blood loss. Aminoglycosides should only be used for prophylaxis in prosthetic surgery and in combination with gram-positive coverage, such as cefazolin. A fourth generation penicillin plus good *Staphylococcus* coverage is an alternative. Any compound adversely affecting coagulation or bleeding should have close monitoring or concomitant vitamin K administration. First and second generation cephalosporins (cefazolin, cefamandole, cefoxitin) are too widely used therapeutically to be preferred drugs for prophylaxis. Ampicillin and nitrofurantoin do not achieve satisfactory serum and tissue levels in the prostate and the former is becoming less effective against many hospital pathogens [89]. TMP-SXT would be acceptable if it covered more nosocomial associated bacteria and could achieve bactericidal levels in the prostate with only single or perioperative doses. The fourth generation of penicillin (piperacillin, mezlocillin) are possibilities for prophylaxis especially in patients with higher likelihood of enterococcus infections. Enterococcal bacteremia may carry a mortality rate as high as 50% [20, 90]. Third generation cephalosporins (single dose) are the preference of many; cefotaxime has an excellent safety record, ceftriaxone has an incredibly long half-life and ceftazidime superior activity against *Pseudomonas*. The latter may be restricted in hospitals because of the possibility of bacterial-resistance occurring if overuse or misuse should occur with this seemingly superb antibiotic.

Again, attention must be paid to the half-life and when the drug is given preoperatively. For example, a drug with a $t_{1/2}$ of 8 h could be safely given 2–3 h preoperatively whereas one with a $t_{1/2}$ of 1 h best be given intravenously in the operating room 30 min before surgery or intramuscularly just before the patient is brought to the operating room. Knowledge of the pharmacokinetics of your prophylaxis choice is simple and essential. The drug should achieve bactericidal levels in urine, serum and target tissue when at all possible at the time of surgery and should cover organisms common to the operative site as well as most nosocomial pathogens.

Conclusion

The contaminated nature of our surgery among potentially infected patients amplifies the importance of preoperative assessment, perioperative antibiotic prophylaxis and postoperative monitoring and care.

Instrumentation and catheterization guidelines must be established and followed in conjunction with rational antimicrobial prescribing to prevent or decrease nosocomial UTIs and infectious complications. Single dose preoperative administration of potent antibiotics that cover common and nosocomial organisms are preferred for genitourinary surgical prophylaxis.

References

1 Centers for Disease Control: National nosocomial infections study report. *Nov.:* 2–14 (1979).

2 Stamm, W.; Martin, S.; Bennett, J.: Session V. Hospital-acquired infections. Epidemiology of nosocomial infections due to gram-negative bacilli: aspects relevant to development and use of vaccines. J. infect. Dis. *136:* suppl., pp. S151–S160 (1977).

3 Fowler, J.: Nosocomial catheter-associated urinary tract infection. Infect. Surg. *2:* 43–53 (1983).

4 Platt, R.; Polk, B.; Murdock, B.; Rosner, B.: Mortality associated with nosocomial urinary tract infection. New Engl. J. Med. *307:* 637–642 (1982).

5 Turck, M.; Stamm, W.: Nosocomial infections of the urinary tract. Am. J. Med. *70:* 651–654 (1981).

6 Madsen, P.; Nielsen, O.: Microflora of urinary tract infections in hospitalized male patients; in Neu, Percival, Antibiotic prophylaxis in surgery: current concepts. Merck Sharp Dohme Int. *29* (1980).

7 Centers for Disease Control: National nosocomial infections study report. Ann. Summary 1978: *7*(1981).

8 Kreger, B.; Craven, D.; Carling, P. et al.: Gram negative bacteremia. III. Reassessment of etiology, epidemiology and ecology in 612 patients. Am. J. Med. *68:* 332–343 (1980).

9 McCabe, W.; Jackson, G.: Gram-negative bacteremia. I. Etiology and ecology. Archs intern. Med. *110:* 845–855 (1962).

10 Kunin, C.; McCormack, R.: Prevention of catheter-induced urinary tract infections by sterile closed drainage. New Engl. J. Med. *274:* 1155–1162 (1966).

11 Garibaldi, R.; Burke, J.; Dickman, M.; et al.: Factors predisposing to bacteriuria during indwelling urethral catheterization. New Engl. J. Med. *291:* 215–218 (1974).

12 Finkelberg, Z.; Kunin, C.: Clinical evaluation of closed urinary drainage systems. J. Am. med. Ass. *207:* 1657–1662 (1969).

13 Nielsen, O.; Maigaard, S.; Frimodt-Moller, N.; Madsen, P.: Prophylactic antibiotics in transurethral prostatectomy. J. Urol. *126:* 60–62 (1981).

14 Childs, S.: Genitourinary surgical prophylaxis. Infect. Surg. *2:* 701–710 (1983).

15 Dellinger, P.: Perioperative antibiotics in urologic surgery. Urol. Clin. N. Am. *3:* 323–331 (1976).

16 Givens, C.; Wenzel, R.: Catheter-associated urinary tract infections in surgical patients? A controlled study on the excess morbidity and costs. J. Urol. *124:* 646–684 (1980).

17 Childs, S.; Wells, W.; Mirelman, S.: Antibiotic prophylaxis for genitourinary surgery in community hospitals. J. Urol. *130:* 305–308 (1983).

18 Krieger, J.; Kaiser, D.; Wenzel, R.: Nosocomial urinary tract infections: secular trends, treatment and economics in a university hospital. J. Urol. *130:* 102–106 (1983).

19 Neu, H.: Urinary tract infections in the 1980's. Semin. Urol. *1:* 130–137 (1983).

20 Childs, S.: Enterococcus in urologic infections. Infect. Surg., Spec. April suppl., pp. 12–14 (1984).

21 Ansell, J.: Some observations on catheter care. J. chron. Dis. *15:* 675–682 (1962).

22 Story, P.: Proteus infections in hospitals. J. Path. Bact. *68:* 55–62 (1954).

23 Edebo, L.; Laurel, G.: Hospital infection of the urinary tract with proteus. Acta path. microbiol. scand. *43:* 93–99 (1958).

24 Brumfitt, W.; Reeves, D.; Faiers, M.; et al.: Antibiotic resistant *E. coli* causing *E. coli* UTI in general practice: relation to fecal flora. Lancet *i:* 315–317 (1971).

25 Stamey, T.: Pathogenesis and treatment of urinary tract infections (Williams & Wilkins, Baltimore 1980).

26 Morris, M.; et al.: The value of prophylactic antibiotics in transurethral prostatic resection. A controlled trial with observations on the origin of postoperative infection. J. Urol. *48:* 479 (1976).

27 Shockman, R.; Messent, D.: The effect of an indwelling catheter on the bacteriology of the male urethra and bladder. Br. med. J. *ii:* 1009 (1954).

28 Garibaldi, T.; Burke, J.; Britt, M.; et al.: Meatal colonization and catheter associated bacteriuria. New Engl. J. Med. *303:* 316 (1980).

29 Schaeffer, A.; Chmiel, J.: Urethral meatal colonization in the pathogenesis of catheter-associated bacteriuria. J. Urol. *130:* 1096–1114 (1983).

30 Maki, D.; Henneken, C.; Phillips, C.; Shaw, W.; Bennett, J.: Nosocomial urinary

tract infections with *Serratia marcescens*. An epidemiologic study. J. infect. Dis. *128:* 579 (1973).
31 McLeod, J.: The hospital urine bottle and bedpan as reservoirs of infection by *Pseudomonas*. Lancet *i:* 394–395 (1958).
32 Maki, D.; Henneken, C.; Bennett, J.: Prevention of catheter associated urinary tract infection, an additional measure. J. Am. med. Ass. *22:* 1270–1271 (1972).
33 Centers for Disease Control: National nosocomial infections study quarterly report: two nosocomial outbreaks of multiple resistant *Proteus rettgeri* infection. Third Quarter *1973:* 10–12 (August 1973).
34 Center for Disease Control: National nosocomial infections study report. Nosocomial *Serratia marcescens* urinary tract infections. First Quarter *1973:* 16–18 (July 1974).
35 Edwards, L.; Cross, A.; Levin, S.; et al.: Outbreak of nosocomial infection with a strain of *Proteus rettgeri:* resistant to many antimicrobials. J. clin. Path. *61:* 41–46 (1974).
36 Echols, R.; Palmer, D.; King, R.; Long, G.: Multidrug-resistant *Serratia marcescens* bacteriuria related to urologic instrumentation. South med. J. *77:* 173–177 (1984).
37 Guze, L.; Beeson, P.: Observations on the reliability and safety of bladder catheterization for bacteriologic study of the urine. New Engl. J. Med. *255:* 474 (1956).
38 Brumfitt, W.; Davies, B.; Rosser, E.: Urethral catheter as a cause of urinary-tract infections in pregnancy and puerperium. Lancet *ii:* 1059 (1961).
39 Marple, C.: Frequency and character of urinary tract infections in an unselected group of women. Ann. intern. Med. *14:* 2220 (1941).
40 Turck, M.; Petersdorf, R.: The role of antibiotics in the prevention of urinary tract infections. J. chron. Dis. *15:* 683 (1962).
41 Stamm, W.: Guidelines for prevention of catheter-associated urinary tract infections. Ann. intern. Med. *82:* 386–390 (1975).
42 Cunha, B.: Nosocomial urinary tract infections. Heart Lung *11:* 545–551 (1982).
43 Thornton, G.; Andriole, V.: Bacteriuria during indwelling catheter drainage. J. Am. med. Ass. *214:* 339–342 (1970).
44 Buddington, W.; Graves, R.: Management of catheter drainage. J. Urol. *62:* 387–393 (1949).
45 Thompson, R.; et al.: Catheter-associated bacteriuria. Failure to reduce attack rates using periodic instillations of a disinfectant into urinary drainage systems. J. Am. med. Ass. *251:* 747–751 (1984).
46 Lindan, R.: The prevention of ascending, catheter-induced infections of the urinary tract. J. chron. Dis. *22:* 321–332 (1969).
47 McGuire, E.: Antibacterial prophylaxis in prostatectomy patients. J. Urol. *111:* 794–798 (1974).
48 Prokocimer, P.; et al.: A prophylaxis by 2 doses of cefotaxime is useful in prostatic surgery. ICAAC Abstr. No. 122 (1983).
49 Korbel, E.; Maher, P.: Use of prophylactic antibiotics in urethral instrumentation. J. Urol. *116:* 744–746 (1976).
50 Shah, P.; Williams, G.; Chaudary, M.: Short-term antibiotic prophylaxis and prostatectomy. Br. J. Urol. *53:* 339–343 (1981).
51 Childs, S.; Mirelman, S.; Wells, W.; Hurst, A.: A comparison of Aztreonam and placebo for genitourinary surgical prophylaxis. ICAAC Abstr. No. 524 (1983).

52 Goldwasser, B.; Bogokowsky, B.; et al.: Prophylactic antimicrobial treatment in transurethral prostatectomy. How long should it be instituted. Urology *XXII:* 136–138 (1983).
53 Goldwasser, B.; Bogokowsky, B.; et al.: Urinary infections following transurethral resection of bladder tumors. Rate and source. J. Urol. *129:* 1123–1124 (1983).
54 Cruse, P.; Foord, R.: Epidemic of postoperative wound infection. A 10-year prospective study of 62,939 wounds. Surg. Clins N. Am. *60:* 27–40 (1980).
55 Flynn, N.; Lawrence, R.: Antimicrobial prophylaxis. Med. Clins N. Am. *63:* 1225–1244 (1979).
56 Burke, J.: Ashley A. Miles and the prevention of infection following surgery. Archs Surg. *119:* 17–19 (1984).
57 Howard, R.: Effect of burn injury, mechanical trauma and operation on host defenses. Surg. Clins N. Am. *59:* 199 (1979).
58 Thomas, M.; et al.: Epidemic of postoperative wound infection associated with ungloved abdominal palpation. Lancet *i:* 1215–1217 (1974).
59 Orr, N.: Is a mask necessary in the operating theater? Ann. R. Coll. Surg. Engl. *63:* 390–392 (1981).
60 Maderazo, M.; Ward, P.: PMN dysfunction in the surgical patient Infect. Surg. *2:* 54–65 (1983).
61 Miles A.: Non-specific defense reactions in bacterial infections. Ann. N.Y. Acad. Sci. *66:* 356–369 (1956).
62 Evans, D.; Miles, A.; Niven, J.: The enhancement of bacterial infections by adrenaline. Br. J. exp. Path. *29:* 20–30 (1948).
63 Miles, A.; Miles, E.; Burke, J.: The value and duration of defense reactions of the skin to the primary lodgement of bacteria. Br. J. exp. Path. *38:* 79–96 (1957).
64 Christou, N.: Anergy testing in surgical patients. Infect. Surg. *2:* 692–700 (1983).
65 Howard, R.: Host defense against infection. I. Curr. Probl. Surg. *17:* 267 (1980).
66 Howard, R.: Host defense against infection. II. Curr. Probl. Surg. *17:* 319 (1980).
67 Mackinnon, A.: Hazardous catheters? J. R. Soc. Med. *77:* 4 (1984).
68 Russo, P.; Packer, M.; Fair, W.: Prophylactic antibiotics in urologic surgery. Semin. Urol. *1:* 155–163 (1983).
69 Centers for Disease Control: Guidelines for prevention of catheter-associated urinary tract infections. Infect Control *2:* 5 (1981).
70 Veterans Administration Ad Hoc: Interdisciplinary advisory committee on antimicrobial drug usage. I. Prophylaxis in surgery. J. Am. med. Ass. *237:* 1003 (1977).
71 Polk, H.; Trachtenberg, L.; Finn, M.: Antibiotic activity in surgical incisions. The basis for prophylaxis in selected operations. J. Am. med. Ass. *244:* 1353 (1980).
72 Madsen, P.; Chaney, M.; Lapinski, E.: NegGram and furadantin in the treatment of infection following transurethral prostatectomy. Acta chir. scand. *129:* 656–661 (1965).
73 Rinker, J.; Witherington, R.: Prophylactic effect of nitrofurantoin (furadantin) in urologic procedures. South. med. J. *62:* 960 (1969).
74 Gross, M.: Use of an antimicrobial agent to prevent complications following transurethral resection of the prostate. Int. Surg. *51:* 475–478 (1969).
75 Miller, A.; Scott, F.; Scott, R.: An evaluation of antibiotics prior to prostatectomy. J. Urol. *92:* 711–713 (1964).

76 Holl, W.; Rous, S.: Is antibiotic prophylaxis worthwhile in patients with transurethral resection of prostate? Urology *XIX:* 43–46 (1982).
77 Burke, J.: The effective period of preventive antibiotic action in experimental incisions and dermal lesions. Surgery *50:* 161 (1961).
78 Goldman, P.; Petersdorf, R.: Prophylactic antibiotics. Controversies give way to guidelines. Drug Ther. *9:* 57 (1979).
79 Ad Hoc Committee of the Committee on Trauma, Division of Medical Sciences, National Academy of Sciences-National Research Council: Postoperative wound infections. The influence of ultraviolet irradiation of the operating room and of various other factors. Ann. Surg. *1:* suppl., p. 160 (1964).
80 Chodak, G.; Plaut, M.: Systemic antibiotics for prophylaxis in urologic surgery. A critical review. J. Urol. *121:* 695–700 (1979).
81 Murphy, D.; Falkiner, F.; Carr, M.; Cafferkey, M.; Gillespie, W.: Septicemia after transurethral prostatectomy. Urology *XXII:* 133–135 (1983).
82 Childs, S.; Wood, P.; Kosola, J.: Antibiotic prophylaxis in genitourinary surgery. Clin. Ther. *4:* Suppl. A (1981).
83 Childs, S.; Wood, P.; Kosola, J.: Antibiotic prophylaxis in genitourinary surgery. A comparison of cefotaxime and cefazolin. Clin. Ther. *5:* supp. A (1982).
84 Childs, S.; Mirelman, S.; Wells, W.: Perioperative use of ceftazidime as a prophylactic agent in transurethral surgery. J. antimicrob. Chemother. *12:* suppl. A, pp. 71–76 (1983).
85 Gibbons, R.; Stark, R.; Correa, R.; Cummings, K.; Mason, J.: The prophylactic use – or misuse – of antibiotics in transurethral prostatectomy. J. Urol. *119:* 381–383 (1978).
86 Weiner, J.; Gibson, G.; Munster, A.: Use of prophylactic antibiotics in surgical procedures. Peer review guidelines as a method for quality assurance. Am. J. Surg. *139:* 348–351 (1980).
87 Jogerst, G.; Dippe, S.: Antibiotic use among medical specialties in a community hospital. J. Am. med. Ass. *245:* 842–846 (1981).
88 Anonymous: Antimicrobial prophylaxis for surgery. Med. lett. *25:* 113–116 (1983).
89 Madsen, P.; Baumueller, A.; Hoyme, U.: Experimental models for determination of antimicrobials in prostatic tissue, interstitial fluid and secretion. Scand. J. infect. Dis. *14:* supp., pp. 145–150 (1978).
90 Klimek, J.; et al.: Enterococcal infections in a large community hospital, with emphasis on bacteremia. Am. J. infect. Control *8:* 58–61 (1980).

S.J. Childs, MD, FACS, Southeastern Research Foundation, Inc.,
P.O. Box 985, Alabaster, AL 35007 (USA)

Antibiot. Chemother., vol. 33, pp. 30–58 (Karger, Basel 1985)

Perioperative Prevention of Infection in Abdominal Surgery

Alan J. Wilson, Colin J.L. Strachan
Brighton General Hospital, Brighton, UK

Introduction

Abdominal operations can be divided into two broad categories, clean and contaminated. Clean operations may be defined as those in which neither the prepared skin nor the operative field contains a significant quantity of pathogenic bacteria. Contaminated operations may be defined as the operative contamination of an initially clean laparotomy when the normal flora of an intra-abdominal organ or the microflora altered by disease or contained within a septic focus is released systemically, intraperitoneally or into the wound.

The experimental work of *Miles* et al. [1] and *Burke* [2] defined the 'decisive period' when agents active against the bacteria released during operation would be most effective. Antibiotics were shown to modify a subsequent infection only if they were administered within 3 or 4 h of bacterial inoculation. The development of a wound infection depends on a balance between the quantity of viable pathogenic bacteria remaining in the wound at the end of an operation [55], the wound environment and the host defence mechanisms, which are still poorly understood. The quantity of pathogenic bacteria depends on the normal resident microflora of the viscera operated upon. This microflora is modified by the pathological state of the specific viscera and the patient's general condition and age. If the total count of viable pathogenic bacteria is greater than 10^5 organisms/ml of fluid then sepsis is likely to occur. The necessity for antimicrobial prophylaxis depends on whether there is a net advantage when the benefits of prophylaxis in preventing septic complications are compared with the potential dangers to the patient and his ecology. In the majority of clean operations, antimicrobial prophylaxis will not be necessary. However, prophylaxis may be useful in apparently clean operations even where the expected rate is as low as 1:50 when such sepsis threatens life itself. For example, graft infection in aortic surgery is rare, but often fatal; whereas the common mild wound infection after appendicectomy does not usually affect the patient's return to work. Therefore, although rates of septic complications give some idea of which patients may benefit from antimicrobial prophylaxis, it is also necessary to consider the possible consequences of sepsis and to identify which factors signify an increased likelihood of subsequent infection.

Incidence of Wound Infections in Particular Operations

One of the major contributions of controlled trials has been the recognition that sepsis rates are often grossly underestimated in uncontrolled prospective and retrospective studies. For example, *Krukowski* et al. [4] in an uncontrolled 5-year prospective study of infection after abdominal surgery recently reported a wound infection rate of only 3.1% after colorectal operations, whereas the controls in previous clinical trials of various antimicrobials have a gross mean sepsis rate of 44% ranging between 20 and 68% [5]. Table I shows the wound infection rates after various operations. The study by *Bröte* [7] of 2,827 operations from a single hospital not using antimicrobial prophylaxis is perhaps the best yardstick to determine which operations have a high sepsis rate and may be usefully controlled by antimicrobial prophylaxis.

General Factors Determining the Rate of Wound Infection

There are certain general factors [10] which contribute to the probability of septic complications. These can be divided into three groups according to the source of infection.

The Patient

Older patients have an increased risk of infection than young patients [6, 8, 11–13]; carriers of staphylococci are at greater risk [14] and a preoperative shower with hexachlorophene reduces wound infection rates in clean surgery [12, 13]; shaving of the skin too early increases

Table I. Wound infection rates in reviews of abdominal surgery

	Ljungqvist [6]	Public Health Laboratory Service [8]	*Wenzel* et al. [9]	*Bröte* [7]
Inguinal hernia, %	1.7	7.3	2.7	1.8
Varicose veins, %	2.7	11.7	–	3.1
Breast operation, %	1.1	15.4	–	3.4
Gastric, %	7.1	8.7	–	16.8
Appendix – simple, %	5.3	6.7	4.4	8.5
Appendix – perforated, %	20.1	43	15	38.7
Colorectal, %	–	–	10	23
Pancreas, %	–	–	–	25
Splenectomy, %	–	–	–	20

wound infection rates [12, 13]; patients anergic to delayed hypersensitivity skin testing [15], which is associated with increasing age, malnourishment [15] and debilitating diseases such as leukaemia, diabetes and advanced solid tumours, are at increased risk of septic complications.

Patient and Hospital Environment

A prolonged preoperative hospitalisation increases wound infection rates in clean surgery from 1.2% for 1 day to 2.1% for 1 week [12, 13]. The large, multibed-type of ward is associated with a higher risk of infection [11].

Surgeon and Theatre Staff

Good surgical technique is undoubtedly one of the main determinants of septic complications. Matters of the surgical scrub, aseptic barriers, skin preparations, wound drapes, drainage of wounds and suture materials have been reviewed in detail by a number of authors [10–12, 112].

Although studies of antimicrobial prophylaxis have concentrated on particular operations, this brief review suggests that there may be patients undergoing operations which do not normally require prophylaxis but who may benefit from antimicrobial prophylaxis, for example mastectomy on an elderly patient after a recent biopsy of the malignant tumour [113]. There is clearly a need to identify these patients and consider controlled clinical trials of antimicrobial prophylaxis.

In abdominal surgery, the bowel is the commonest source of pathogens. A knowledge of the normal bacterial microflora and the influence of the pathological state on this microflora is valuable in determining the quantity and species of bacteria likely to be encountered and the selection of appropriate antibiotics for prophylaxis.

Influence of Pathological States on the Normal Microflora of the Bowel

Solid viscera, peritoneal cavity, blood vessels and renal tract are normally sterile. The gastro-intestinal tract contains a variable quantity of bacteria throughout its length. In the oesophagus, stomach and proximal small bowel, bacteria are relatively sparse and seldom exceed 10^5/ml of aspirate. The normal oesophagus contains a flora similar to that found in the oropharynx [16, 17] where *Streptococcus viridans* is the commonest aerobic isolate. *Haemophilus influenzae, Neisseria catarrhalis, Klebsiella pneumoniae* and *Streptococcus* spp. have also been isolated from the oesophagus of normal volunteers. *Peptococcus* is the commonest anaerobic isolate followed in frequency by *Peptostreptococcus, Bacteroides melanogenicus* and *Bacteroides fragilis.* The anaerobic organisms, except *B. fragilis* (which was isolated from 8% of patients with carcinoma of the oesophagus [16]), are sensitive to penicillin. The same frequency of bacterial isolates occurs in patients with carcinoma of the oesophagus, but presumably the total viable count of organisms is higher in this and any other condition which obstructs or damages the mucosa of the oesophagus. One study is underway to determine the effect of irrigation of the oesophagus with metronidazole [17].

The normal stomach contains bacteria at concentrations of 10^2–10^5/ml of aspirate and acts as a barrier to the further passage of ingested micro-organisms. Its effectiveness as a barrier is primarily dependent on the secretion of hydrochloric acid [59] and the total viable bacterial count is proportional to the pH [59, 61] and degree of stasis [60]. The normal microflora consists of streptococci, aerobic lactobacilli, diphtheroids and fungi [18]. But in patients with hypochlorhydria the stomach is invaded by *Escherichia coli, Klebsiella* spp. and *Proteus* spp. in combination with penicillin-sensitive anaerobes such as *Peptostreptococcus* and *B. melanogenicus* [59, 61, 64].

The concentration of bacteria in the normal proximal small bowel is 10^2–10^4/ml mainly because of the gastric barrier to ingested microorganisms [19]. In the presence of gastric hypochlorhydria, inhibition of normal motility, blind loops after various operative procedures and diseases of the small bowel wall there is a considerable increase in the population of the resident flora and an influx of coliforms and penicillin-resistant obligate anaerobes ranging from 10^6 to 10^8 viable organisms/ml [18]. The normal resident flora of the small bowel increases distally such that 10^4–10^7 organisms/ml exist in the terminal ileum [19].

The colon contains between 10^{11} and 10^{12} organisms/ml of faeces and most notably the ratio of anaerobes to aerobes is between 100 and 1,000:1. There are between 200 and 400 bacterial species present in a single specimen of faeces. The commonest anaerobes are *B. fragilis, Eubacteria, Bifidobacteria, Clostridia* and anaerobic cocci. The aerobes are *E. coli* and other coliforms, enterococci and bacillus species. Despite this enormously diverse bacterial flora, the commonest isolates from septic complications of colorectal surgery are *E. coli* and *B. fragilis.* Nature has been kind to the surgeon contemplating antibiotic therapy.

The importance of anaerobes in septic complications has become widely recognised only in the past decade [20]. The pathogenicity of *B. fragilis* depends on a synergism with aerobic organisms such as *E. coli* [3] and the presence of a polysaccharide capsule which seems to potentiate abscess formation [21], possibly by inhibiting phagocytosis [22].

Although this section has only considered the gastro-intestinal tract there are examples of abdominal viscera which are normally sterile becoming infected as a result of structural damage or obstruction. These will be considered separately in the following sections.

Review of Controlled Trials of Antimicrobial Prophylaxis

In reviewing the results of controlled trials of antimicrobial prophylaxis we have begun with appendicitis. Although this disease has a well-defined natural history and a limited number of septic complications, there are still problems inherent in the interpretation of the maze of trials involving the use of antimicrobial prophylactic therapy.

Appendicitis

In 1982 there were 154 cases of death from appendicitis reported in the returns of the Registrar General for England and Wales. Although appendicitis is now a rare cause of death, it continues to cause a significant morbidity from septic complications. These include intraperitoneal and pelvic abscesses, generalised peritonitis, septicaemia, wound infection and the later complications of incisional hernia and bowel obstruction secondary to adhesions. Postoperative intraperitoneal abscess occurs in about 2% of patients with acute appendicitis [24] and 10% of patients operated on for perforated appendicitis [23, 26].

Wound infection is the commonest septic complication. The overall incidence varies considerably between different series. For example, rates of 20% and 0% [36] have been reported following removal of a normal appendix in patients not receiving antibiotics.

Factors Influencing the Reported Incidence of Wound Infection

The reported incidence of wound infection depends on a number of factors: *Definition of Wound Infection. Ljungqvist* [6] defined wound infection as 'a clear collection of pus which empties itself spontaneously or after incision'. A large proportion of authors of the publications which will be subsequently discussed use a modification of this definition. Some include all serosanguineous discharges from the wound [45] whilst others depend either on the results of bacteriological culture for classification [33, 48] or the need for repeated dressings [26]. Certain authors graded wound infection and thus produced a more concise definition [34, 45].

Stringency of Follow-Up. 60–65% of wound infections only become apparent after the 7th postoperative day [45] when the patient has usually been discharged from hospital [48, 49]. Careful follow-up by an unbiased observer is therefore necessary to assess the effectiveness of antimicrobial prophylaxis. Follow-up by telephone or questionnaire [30] is open to criticism and any paper presenting data that all wound infections had occurred by the 3rd postoperative day [32] is clearly suspect, particularly if certain antimicrobials merely delay the presentation of wound infections [44]. Indeed this raises the point that with antimicrobial prophylaxis there may be a shift in the incidence of major sepsis from the hospital to the community. Trials of antibiotic prophylaxis must take this into consideration in evaluating the benefits of treatment.

Variations in Risk Factors within the Total Group. The pathological state of the appendix is the most powerful predictor of septic complications. Wound infection is about four times more likely if the appendix is gangrenous or perforated compared to normal or merely inflamed.

Obese [39, 54] and old [33] patients have a greater risk of developing wound infection. This is related to an increased incidence of gangrene and perforation, presumably due to a delay in the diagnosis of these difficult patients.

Differences in surgical technique also affect the likelihood of intraperitoneal abscess and wound infection. Some of these have been identified and include the size of the wound, whether the abdominal wall muscle is cut [33], the use of diathermy [12, 13], abdominal drains [25], protection of the wound edges by swabs soaked in antiseptic solution [38], the length of time the operation takes [51], whether or not the appendix stump is buried and routine lavage of the pelvic cavity with saline or antiseptic solutions [4].

Bacteriology of Appendicitis

E. coli and *B. fragilis* are the commonest bacteria isolated from peritoneal swabs [26, 48, 50], the appendix [33] and the pus of wound infections. The detection of bacteria depends on the pathological state of the appendix [33, 51] and on the care taken over the collection, transport, culture and identification of the bacteria. In a study of 112 children [50] presenting with perforated appendicitis, 89% of peritoneal swabs taken at operation grew bacteria and of these 74% grew a mixture of aerobic and anaerobic organisms. Anaerobic bacteria were isolated either alone or in combination with an aerobic bacteria in 88% of peritoneal swabs and 91% of wound exudates. The commonest aerobes were *E. coli* (57%), various streptococci and *Pseudomonas aeruginosa* (9%) and the commonest anaerobes were *B. fragilis* (54%), *B. melaninogenicus* (21%) and *Peptostreptococcus* spp. There was a mean of 4.45 bacterial isolates per peritoneal swab. The same distribution of bacterial species was isolated from infected wounds. Thus *E. coli* removed from the inhibitory interactions of the bowel lumen becomes a virulent pathogen in the wound.

The risk of subsequent wound infection increases if bacteria are

Table II. Randomised controlled trials of topical antiseptics and antibiotics in appendicectomy

	Total number of patients analysed	Wound infection, %		p	Reference
		no treatment	treatment		
Povidone-iodine[1]	221	10	12	NS	48
Povidone-iodine	300	16	8	0.03	33
Povidone-iodine	236	24	24	NS	27
'Savlon' solution	252	10	10	NS	24
'Polybactrin'	300	16	9	0.06	33
Ampicillin 1 g[2, 3]	246	10	3	0.05	24
Ampicillin 0.5 g	200	16	3	0.01	40
Ampicillin 0.5 g	150	24	9	0.02	39
Ampicillin 1 g	374	9	0.1	0.01	46
Ampicillin 1 g	130	24	3	0.01	47

1 Povidone-iodine spray applied to wound at end of operation.
2 Ampicillin powder used in all trials.
3 Ampicillin powder was effective for all pathological states of the appendix.

isolated from a perioperative wound swab [26, 33, 48]. However, the presence of bacteria in the wound at the end of an operation does not inevitably lead to wound infection. In one study [48] although *Bacteroides* spp. were isolated from the intraoperative wounds of 47 patients, only 12 patients developed a wound infection. *Streptococcus milleri* has recently been cultured in appendicectomy wounds and is related to a high risk of sepsis [*Tanner,* personal communication].

Results of Clinical Trials of Antimicrobial Prophylaxis

Topical Agents. The results of trials of topical antiseptics and antibiotics are shown in table II. Although one trial [33] showed a significant benefit for patients who had povidone-iodine spray applied to the wound at the end of the operation, two other trials [27, 48] were unable to support this conclusion. On the other hand the application of ampicillin powder consistently reduced the rate of wound infection for all pathological states of the appendix.

Table III. Randomised controlled trials of metronidazole given alone

Dose	Route	Timing	Total number of patients analysed	Wound infection, %		p	Reference
				control	treatment		
0.5 mg	i.v.	preop.	100	24	2	0.002	37
1 g	p.r.	preop. + 2 days	90	15	5	–	35
1 g[1]	p.r.	preop.	278	11	1	0.005	36
1 g	p.r.	preop. + 2 doses	187	8	5	NS	34
1 g	p.r.	preop. + 4 doses	127	30	21	0.1	44
1 g[1]	p.r.	preop. + 5 doses	375	24	12	0.01	27

[1] All groups of pathological state affected.

Systemic Antibiotics. Metronidazole (table III) given alone either as a single preoperative dose or continuing with additional postoperative doses is an effective agent in preventing wound infection. However, it is notable that two trials [34, 44] were unable to demonstrate a significant effect. In the largest trial [27], it was possible to demonstrate that Flagyl significantly reduced wound infection for all pathological states of the appendix. There was no evidence in any of these trials that a short course of metronidazole caused toxic side effects. In addition, it has been shown that Flagyl is more effective than povidone-iodine spray in preventing wound infections [49].

Cephalosporins (table IV) given alone seem to be effective in reducing the incidence of wound infection, but only two trials [28, 51] of cephalosporins with a limited range of activity against anaerobes demonstrated a conclusive benefit. One trial using cefotaxime, which has an extended spectrum of activity against anaerobic organisms, demonstrated a significant benefit against patients receiving Flagyl alone [45].

Finally, three trials have examined whether agents active against both aerobic and anaerobic organisms might be more effective than agents only active against aerobic or anaerobic organisms. *Morris* [44] demonstrated that cefazolin plus metronidazole was more effective than when either agent was given alone. *Lau* et al. [45] demonstrated that cefotaxime and Flagyl were more effective than Flagyl given alone but that cefotaxime was as effective as the combination of agents. It

Table IV. Randomized controlled trials of cephalosporins in appendicitis

Drug	Dose	Route	Timing	Total number of patients analysed[2]	Wound infection, % control	Wound infection, % treated	p	Reference
Cephaloridine	50 mg/kg	i.m.	preop. + 2 days	139	12	1.4	0.02	28
Cefoxitin	2 g	i.v.	preop. + 2 doses	120	7	1.5	NS	31
Cefoxitin	1 g	i.v.	preop. + 2 doses	103	10	0	0.05	30
Cefazolin	1 g	i.m.	preop.	123	27	17	NS	29
Cefamandole	2 g	i.v.	preop. + 1 day	91	13	2	0.05	51
Cefazolin	1 g	i.v.	preop. + 4 doses	131	30	20	0.08	44
Cefotaxime[1]	1 g	i.v.	preop.	205	30	13	0.01	45

[1] Control group treated with Flagyl.
[2] Excludes patients in other arms of the trial.

might be argued that a potent antibiotic such as cefotaxime should be reserved as a therapeutic agent for the treatment of serious established infections. *Busuttil* et al. [51] found that the addition of carbenicillin did not reduce the rate of wound infection compared with cephamandole given alone.

Perforated Appendicitis

When perforation or gangrene is present, prophylaxis becomes 'treatment'. This condition still presents problems in the prevention of intraperitoneal abscess and wound infection. In one trial [45], a quarter of patients treated with cefotaxime still suffered a wound infection although this was approximately half that of a group of patients who had only been treated with Flagyl. In both groups of patients, the antibiotics were continued for 5 days after operation. Two trials [26] have demonstrated that the application of topical ampicillin powder significantly reduces wound infection and that there is no benefit if wound closure is delayed until the 5th day. *Berne* et al. [42] purported to show that clindamycin and gentamicin given for at least 5 days were significantly better than cephamandole and cefaperazone. However, the dosage of the cephalosporins was probably below therapeutic levels.

Other End-Point Evaluation in Trials

In none of the trials reviewed was there a death from sepsis. None of the trials demonstrated a significant reduction in the relatively rare complication of intraperitoneal abscess. In a 'pre-anaerobe' trial by *Magarey* et al. [25] there was no difference in the number of days off work despite an increased rate of wound infection in the group with intraperitoneal drains. In the trial by *Foster* et al. [27], patients treated with Flagyl returned to work 3 days earlier than the placebo group despite large differences in wound infection rates.

There was no difference in the mean duration of hospital stay in the trial by *Berne* et al. [42] but *Foster* et al. [27] and *Busuttil* et al. [51] found that hospital stay was significantly reduced by the use of antimicrobial prophylaxis. Delayed primary suture of wounds in patients with perforated appendicitis increased the duration of hospital stay [26]. The number of visits by district nurses was reduced for patients receiving Flagyl compared to placebo or povidone-iodine spray [27].

Conclusions

In a survey of current UK surgical practice (1980) in the prophylaxis of infection after appendicectomy [52], 43% of surgeons never used prophylactic systemic antibiotics in uncomplicated acute appendicitis. 61% sometimes used a topical agent (63% used povidone-iodine and 6% ampicillin powder). 77% of surgeons sometimes drained the peritoneal cavity.

There still seems to be considerable ignorance and indifference when surgeons select their prophylactic regime for patients presenting with acute appendicitis and its sequelae.

Recommendations

If the patient presents with localised right iliac fossa pain it would seem that only anti-anaerobe cover is necessary. This can be ideally and cost-effectively provided by a 1-gram suppository of metronidazole given at least 1–2 h before surgery to achieve adequate blood and tissue levels. The wound should be closed by primary suture without drainage after infected fluid has been sucked out of the pelvis.

For cases of a gangrenous or perforated appendix, systemic administration of antibiotics active against aerobes and anaerobes should be commenced immediately upon diagnosis. The treatment should be reviewed at 48–72 h in the light of the culture of a sample of preoperative pus. The anti-anaerobe would be either metronidazole or tinidazole (the latter has a longer half-life) or clindamycin (which has recently been condemned in the UK for its adverse reactions). The anti-aerobe spectrum is more difficult. We have found that the perioperative culture of *S. faecalis* and *S. milleri* was associated with a particularly high incidence of subsequent sepsis. Although gentamicin and ampicillin have been used in the past, these agents are toxic and allergenic when used in the continued treatment regimen which may be necessary for perforated and gangrenous appendicitis. Cefuroxime, cefotetan and cefotaxime provide excellent cover, except for certain streptococci. Mezlocillin and piperacillin have a broad spectrum of activity, but again should perhaps be reserved for life-threatening sepsis.

Many extrovert surgeons like the 'efficacious' dark brown of povidone iodine spray or the purity of white antibiotic powder billowing into the overhead lighting system, but others closer to the agar plate are aware of the potential ecological disaster of topical antibiotic powders. Preoperative intra-incisional injection is a novel method which may be less liable to provoke resistant strains.

Problems Concerning Trials of Antimicrobial Prophylaxis

Before considering the larger and more complex field of colorectal surgery we shall indicate some of the problems of clinical trials using appendicitis as an example. Antimicrobial agents may be administered to prevent wound infection by the topical or systemic route. Comparative trials of antimicrobial prophylaxis present certain problems concerning randomisation procedures, the distinction between protocol deviation and violation, and the subsequent end-point evaluation. For example, a randomisation procedure which used the patient's date of birth [30] will give a preconception of the allotted treatment, whilst selection by envelopes in theatre is always open to manipulation. Trials of topical application of antiseptics and antibiotics cannot be blinded because there is no placebo which may not affect local wound factors predisposing to infection.

Clinical trials of antimicrobial prophylaxis may compare either policies of management or the effectiveness of a particular antibiotic in preventing infection due to certian pathogens. The former approach is orientated towards the patient and might include evaluation of the time taken to return to work, loss of earnings, postoperative pain and inconvenience and the cost of hospitalisation. The only exclusions in such a trial might be patients who are known to be allergic to the antibiotic. The second approach concentrates on the rate of infection and demands certain exclusions including such retrospective protocol violations as inappropriate administration of the antibiotic. The more exclusions then the more limited are the conclusions and the less the application to actual clinical practice.

Colonic and Rectal Surgery

Many reviews and tabulations of the results of clinical trials have been published [56–59] and the reader is referred to these for further information.

Development of Effective Antimicrobial Prophylaxis through Randomised Clinical Trials

In 1969, *Sellwood* et al. [73] demonstrated in a randomised control trial that a combination of neomycin, bacitracin and nystatin given orally for 48 h before surgery resulted in a significant suppression of the viable count of faecal bacterial species including bacteroides, coliforms, streptococci and clostridia. On the other hand phthalylsulphathiazole given orally alone did not significantly reduce these species of bacteria. The incidence of infections was 62% for phthalylsulphathiazole and 21% for the combination of antibiotics.

Between 1970 and 1979 there was an enormous effort to determine the most effective antimicrobial propyhlactic regime. In 1973 *Nicholls* et al. [74] demonstrated that neomycin 1 g plus erythromycin base 1 g orally given in three doses in a 10-hour period before operation resulted in a significant reduction in the colonic microflora including the *Enterobacteriaceae* and *Bacteroides* spp. In a subsequent randomised control trial [75], this regime versus mechanical bowel preparation alone was shown to be effective in reducing the incidence of wound infection from 35 to 9% and more importantly it showed that the incidence of intraperitoneal abscess, anastomotic leak and septicaemia were also significantly reduced.

The majority of the infections were due to a mixture of aerobic and anaerobic organisms: *B. fragilis* was isolated from 6 out of 8 septicaemic patients in the control group [76, 77]. Collection of faeces at 7 and 14 days postoperatively showed no increase of antibiotic-resistant gram-negative bacilli, staphylococci or fungi [76].

Tetracycline is an effective substitute for erythromcyin [77] although it is notable that tetracycline inhibits only about 40% of *B. fragilis* in vitro.

Kanamycin 1 g orally (which like neomycin is not absorbed in significant amounts from the bowel lumen) and metronidazole 200 mg orally (which is absorbed systemically and is only active against anaerobic organisms) given 6-hourly for 3 preoperative days is an equally effective regime in reducing the incidence of wound infection and reducing the colonic aerobic and anaerobic microflora [78]. Neomycin 1 g orally and Flagyl 200 mg orally 8-hourly for 2 days preoperatively significantly reduced wound infection rate, perineal sepsis after abdominoperineal resection, septicaemia and anastomotic leak [79].

Neomycin alone is not effective in reducing septic complications compared with placebo [77] and neither does it reduce *E. coli* species in the colon [80]. *Arabi* et al. [80] also found that metronidazole alone had no effect on the quantity of viable aerobes and anaerobes within the large bowel, but combinations of neomycin and Flagyl significantly reduced both aerobic and anaerobic bacteria. In addition, they found an increase in the number of resistant strains of *E. coli* and *S. faecalis* during treatment with neomycin. Mechanical bowel preparation alone does not alter the anaerobic microflora of the large bowel [109, 110].

Systemic Antimicrobial Prophylaxis

One of the earliest control trials of systemic prophylaxis was by *Polk and Lopez-Mayor* [82] who demonstrated that cephaloridine 1 g i.m. immediately before operation followed by two postoperative doses reduced wound infection rates from 15 to 4% in colorectal operations. In retrospect this result is surprising in view of the weak activity of cephaloridine against anaerobic bacteria [111]. However, it confirmed that a very short course of antibiotic prophylaxis is all that may be required in preventing wound infection and other septic complications. *Stone* et al. [83] demonstrated that cefazolin 1 g i.m. which has relatively greater activity against anaerobes than cephaloridine [111] was an effective agent in reducing wound infections but only if it was administered either 8–12 h or 1 h preoperatively. This trial provided confirmation of the experimental work of *Miles and Burke* [1, 2]. Recent studies on the effect of second- and third-generation cephalosporins and cephamycins show the production of resistant *Enterobacteriaceae* by cefoxitin, cefaperazone and moxalactam.

Subsequent Development of Clinical Trials in Antimicrobial Prophylaxis

Once it had been shown that antimicrobial prophylaxis was an effective agent in reducing the septic complications of colorectal surgery, clinical trials attempted to determine a number of facts including the effectiveness of different combinations of antibiotics, the value of single agents particularly those effective against anaerobic organisms, the length of time that antibiotics need to be administered and the side effects of different antibiotic treatments.

Antibiotics which are specifically active against anaerobes and have been shown to be effective prophylactic agents in colorectal surgery include erythromycin [75], lincomycin [84], tetracycline [77] and metronidazole [85, 97, 103]. In all of these trials an agent active against aerobes was also administered.

Single agents active only against aerobes have in general not proved to be efficacious [77, 81] but agents used alone against anaerobes do reduce wound infection rates and other septic complications. Lincomycin 600 mg preoperatively and for 5 days postoperatively [87] significantly reduced wound infection rates and the incidence of septicaemia. However, lincomycin is associated with a particularly high incidence of pseudomembranous colitis and is no longer recommended. Doxycycline, which is active against anaerobes and some intestinal aerobes, administered preoperatively and 5 days postoperatively is effective for most septic complications [88], Flagyl given preoperatively and for 5 days postoperatively reduces sepsis rates [89] although it did not reduce perineal sepsis after abdominoperineal resection of the rectum.

The results of these trials using single agents effective against only anaerobes might suggest that an agent active against aerobes is unnecessary. A number of trials have been performed to test this hypothesis. These trials have produced conflicting results. Two trials have demonstrated the apparent necessity for combination therapy. *Hansell* et al. [94] demonstrated that the omission of kanamycin in a regime consisting of kanamycin and Flagyl resulted in an increase in wound infection rates. This is supported by another trial which showed a beneficial effect if cefuroxime and Flagyl were compared to Flagyl alone [90]. In contradiction to these results *Mitchell* et al. [91] found that the addition of a single dose of cefuroxime 1.5 mg i.v. to a single preoperative dose of Flagyl 500 mg i.v. did not affect the sepsis rate. *Morris* et al. [92] were unable to demonstrate any benefit if gentamicin 160 mg i.v. was added to Flagyl 500 mg i.v. administered in three doses. There would seem to be a need for further clinical trials in examining this question.

Route of Administration of Antibiotics

There are certain advantages in using the systemic route rather than the oral route. *Keighley* et al. [93] compared kanamycin and Flagyl orally versus the same drugs given intravenously preoperatively. Although the oral drugs which were given for 2 days preoperatively reduced the colonic concentrations of aerobic and anaerobic organisms whereas the intravenous drugs given just prior to operation did not reduce the bacterial count, the incidence of abdominal sepsis was significantly lower in the systemic group (6.5%) than in the oral therapy group (32%). In addition, 15 out of 17 patients with septic complications in the oral therapy group had resistant bacteria in the colon at the time of operation and an increased incidence of pseudomembranous colitis. In contradiction, *Hansell* et al. [94] showed no difference in septic complications between oral and intravenous kanamycin and Flagyl. However, 15 out of 32 patients receiving oral kanamycin became colonised by kanamycin-resistant organisms during the 3-day preoperative period of prophylaxis.

These results might suggest that tissue levels of antibiotics are more important than a quantitative reduction of the bacterial content of the gut prior to surgery. This is not an easy problem to investigate for, although *Keighley* et al. [93] demonstrated no reduction in the anaerobic microflora after a single intravenous dose of kanamycin and Flagyl, *Dion* et al. [95] demonstrated in a careful study of patients receiving a standard mechanical bowel preparation plus neomycin, that *Bacteroides* spp. were equally reduced in the colon by Flagyl given either orally for 2 preoperative days or intravenously 1 h prior to surgery.

The problem of oral versus systemic is compounded by the results of a trial by *Coppa* et al. [102] which demonstrated that the addition of three doses of intravenous cefoxitin 1 g to the standard neomycin plus erythromycin regime of *Nicholls* et al. [74] significantly reduced wound infection rates. However, it is noteworthy that in the subsequent discussion of this paper *Condon* pointed out that the infection rate of 18% in the control group was unduly high and the preoperative oral regimen was not identical to *Nicholls'* regimen.

Length of Time for Preoperative Antimicrobial Prophylaxis

Stone [83] has reported that cephamandole is equally effective if given either as a three-dose perioperative regime or as a 3-day course of preoperative therapy resulting in a considerable saving of hospital costs. *Higgins* et al. [98] reported that a single preoperative dose is as effective as a 5-day course of cotrimoxazole and Flagyl. However, *Eykyn* et al. [96] although they obtained good results from a single preoperative dose of Flagyl followed by two postoperative doses found three wound infections which gave rise to *Bacteroides* spp., whereas in most trials which have used a prolonged postoperative course of Flagyl there were no reported infections caused by *Bacteroides* spp. [85, 97].

These results seem to suggest that a single preoperative systemic dose of antibiotics followed by two further doses postoperatively may be all that is required for effective antimicrobial prophylaxis. Theoretically, a short course of antibiotics is less likely to give rise to antibiotic-resistant strains of bacteria.

Alternative Antibiotics

A number of trials have compared different antibiotics with similar spectra of activity. A single dose of ticarcillin and three doses of cephalothin are equally effective [99]. The extended spectrum of cefoxitin [86] is equally effective as doxycycline [100]. Kanamycin and cephamandole [101] are equally effective when added to Flagyl in preventing septic complications.

Future of Trials of Antimicrobial Prophylaxis

There is now no doubt that antimicrobial prophylaxis is a valuable and mandatory adjunct to surgery of the large bowel. It has been considered unethical to withhold antibiotic prophylaxis for colorectal operations for the last decade [104, 108]. It is therefore surprising that in 1979 in a survey of the Veterans Administration Chiefs of Surgery, 16% omitted antibiotic prophylaxis in colorectal cases [104]. In Scotland [105] in 1982, 95% of surgeons used prophylaxis for colorectal surgery although 19% used oral regimes lasting more than 4 preoperative days and 14% failed to use agents active against anaerobic organisms. In Wessex, UK [106] all but 1 of 42 surgeons used preoperative prophylactic antibiotics and only 1 did not provide cover for anaerobic organisms. Neomycin orally and cephradine systemically were the favoured anti-aerobic agents and Flagyl the commonest anti-anaerobic agent.

There are still problems concerning antimicrobial prophylaxis. Firstly, although it has been clearly demonstrated that prophylaxis reduces the incidence of major complications such as anastomotic leakage and septicaemia, it is still conceivable that these complications may be secondary to gross wound sepsis. If wound sepsis could be eradicated by methods other than antibiotics then septicaemia and anastomotic leakage might also be reduced.

If untreated control groups are no longer considered ethical then the number of patients required in trials rises dramatically. About 1,000 patients are needed in a trial to demonstrate a difference of 10% at a probability level of 5% with a 90% degree of certainty that the result is correct. To achieve these numbers, multicentre trials are necessary and with them the attendant rise in costs and manpower needed to organise such trials. Finally, when the benefits of antimicrobial prophylaxis become small as measured by infection rates then the risks of prophylaxis may outweigh the apparent benefits. This is well illustrated by a recent trial in which mezlocillin and Flagyl were compared with cefuroxime and Flagyl [107]. 96 patients were randomised to receive three doses of either set of drugs. Severe wound sepsis occurred in 6% of patients receiving mezlocillin and 16% of patients receiving cefuroxime (not significant). Minor wound sepsis occurred in 24% receiving mezlocillin and 11% receiving cefuroxime (not significant), but the addition of all septic complications produced a significant benefit for patients receiving cefuroxime. However, 13% of patients receiving cefuroxime and 0% receiving mezlocillin developed diarrhoea. *Pseudomonas* were more commonly isolated after cefuroxime than mezlocillin and *Staphylococcus albus* after mezlocillin. In addition, the concentration of antibiotics administered may have been inadequate to maintain serum and tissue concentrations. The problem now is how to balance the risks and benefits of antimicrobial prophylaxis in large bowel surgery.

Recommendations

Table V shows the wide variety of antibiotic combinations commonly used in various countries. There seems to be little evidence that any particular combination is more effective.

In emergency colorectal surgery, the oral antibiotic regimens are

Table V. Commonly used antibiotics for prophylaxis in colorectal surgery

Country	Primary activity	
	anti-aerobe	anti-anaerobe
USA	neomycin gentamicin 2nd generation cephalosporins cefamandole, cephamycin, cefoxitin	erythromycin clindamycin
Canada	aminoglycoside cephalosporin	metronidazole
UK	kanamycin gentamicin tobramycin cefuroxime cefamandole also: tetracycline lavage in a few centres	metronidazole tinidazole
Scandinavia	cefoxitin	doxycycline metronidazole tinidazole
Australia	kanamycin cefamandole	tinidazole metronidazole

obviously ineffective. The toxic side effects of the aminoglycosides and the necessity of serum assay make cover requiring more than 24 h less appealing now that broad-spectrum cephalosporins are available, e.g., cefotaxime, cefotetan or perhaps latamoxef if the latter proves to be free of the reported bleeding tendency in the elderly. Antibiotics should probably be given for 48 h if there has been faecal soiling of the peritoneal cavity and then reassessed in the light of sensitivity reports. The selection of an appropriate antibiotic may soon be possible at an earlier stage when gas chromatography, carbon-labelling techniques or even an immunofluorescent 'sandwich' technique using monoclonal antibodies is commercially available.

Table VI. Effect of pathological state of the stomach on the incidence of wound infection [60]

	Number of patients	With growth at operation, %	Wound infection, %
Simple duodenal ulcer	18	17	0
Bleeding duodenal ulcer	12	100	33
Pyloric stenosis	9	89	11
Carcinoma of stomach	4	100	25
Gastric ulcer	6	83	16

Gastroduodenal Surgery

Identification of Patients at Risk of Sepsis

The rate of septic complications following gastroduodenal surgery is proportional to the quantitative bacterial counts of gastric aspirate [61], the pH of gastric aspirate [61, 64] and the pathological state of the stomach [60]. Table VI shows the influence of pathological state on the incidence of wound infection and the percentage of patients with a significant perioperative isolate of viable bacteria.

Patients are likely to develop septic complications if the preoperative gastric aspirate contains more than 5×10^6 organisms/ml. *Gatehouse* et al. [61] found a wound infection rate of 94% in this group of patients. In addition, if the pH is greater than 4 as occurs in bleeding duodenal ulcer, gastric ulcer, carcinoma of the stomach or preoperative treatment with a histamine-2 antagonist the risks of septic complications are greater. However, in the acid environment of perforated duodenal ulcers 70% of patients have a sterile peritonitis [62].

Bacteriology

The commonest organisms isolated from gastric aspirates and wound infections of such patients are *E. coli*, *Klebsiella* spp., *Proteus*, usually mixed with anaerobes including streptococci, peptostreptococci and *B. melanogenicus* [59–61, 64]. The majority of anaerobes are penicillin-sensitive although *B. fragilis* is occasionally isolated from patients with carcinoma of the stomach.

Results of Controlled Trials

Randomised controlled trials have demonstrated the effectiveness of cephamandole 2 g i.v. 1 h preoperatively plus two postoperative doses [63], cephaloridine 2 g i.v. preoperatively plus one postoperative dose [66] and cefuroxime 1.5 g i.v. preoperatively [64] in preventing wound infections and in the last trial in reducing intraperitoneal abscess formation in high-risk gastric surgery. The untreated control group in this trial had 35% wound infections, 29% abscess formation, 21% septicaemia and the treated group had only 7% of patients who developed a septic complication, all of which were wound infections. In the third arm of this trial, cefuroxime 1.5 g intra-incisional at the end of the operation significantly reduced wound infection, but did not alter the incidence of other septic complications.

Recommendations

Second-generation cephalosporin or mezlocillin given in a single dose are suitable antibiotics for the prophylaxis of upper gastro-intestinal surgery. They are probably only necessary if the bowel is opened during the operation.

Abdominal Aortic Surgery

The walls of abdominal aortic aneurysms are often infected. Bacteria can be cultured from aneurysmal contents in 38% of ruptured aneurysms, 13% of symptomatic and 9% of asymptomatic aneurysms [69]. About 66% of these cases culture a pure growth of staphylococci whilst the remainder culture *Enterobacteriaceae* spp. and anaerobic bacteria [68]. In a randomised control trial [68] cefazolin 1 g i.v. preoperatively plus four postoperative doses significantly reduced the incidence of wound infection in patients undergoing a variety of arterial surgical procedures. This benefit was particularly significant for patients undergoing abdominal aortic surgery where wound infections were as high as 12%. This trial also demonstrated that there was a significantly greater incidence of infection after hexachlorophene-ethanol skin preparation in comparison with povidone-iodine preparation.

In a non-randomised prospective study of 245 abdominal aortic aneurysms repaired, there was a graft infection rate of 7.5% if no prophylactic antibiotics were given versus 0.7% if cloxacillin was administered [67]. Inlay grafts seem to be at particularly high risk of infection.

Although there is still doubt as to the pathogenesis of aortoenteric fistulas [70, 71], it would seem that of the 38% which occur within 12 months of aortic surgery [71] the majority are caused by graft infection at the time of surgery. At least 74% of aortoenteric fistulas are infected and therefore all these patients will also require antibiotics against staphylococci, *Enterobacteriaceae* and anaerobic bacteria. The majority of patients with infected grafts will require complete resection of the graft and extra-anatomic bypass grafting.

Although there is no conclusive evidence from controlled clinical trials that prophylactic antibiotics reduce the incidence of graft infection, the results of these studies seem to indicate that prophylactic antibiotics should always be administered in patients undergoing abdominal aortic surgery.

Recommendations

Perioperative antibiotic cover is still rather empirical. The second-generation cephalosporins have not been surpassed by third-generation or any other new products on the horizon. It seems that as the pseudomonas or gram-negative end of the nucleus is improved there is a loss of efficacy against *Staphylococcus aureus.* Bacteriological culture of the wall of the aorta may require the addition of an agent active against the *Enterobacteriaceae.* Cefamandole or cefuroxime or cefazolin would be suitable antibiotics for initial prophylaxis.

References

1 Miles, A.A.; Miles, E.M.; Burke, J.F.: The value and duration of defence reactions of the skin to the primary lodgement of bacteria. Br. J. exp. Path. *38:* 79–96 (1957).

2 Burke, J.F.: The effective period of preventive antibiotic action in experimental incisions and dermal lesions. Surgery *50:* 161–168 (1961).

3 Kelly, M.J.: Wound infection: a controlled clinical and experimental demonstration of synergy between aerobic *(Escherichia coli)* and anaerobic *(Bacteroides fragilis)* bacteria. Ann. R. Coll. Surg. *62:* 52–59 (1980).

4 Krukowski, Z.H.; Stewart, M.P.M.; Alsayer, H.M.; Matheson, N.A.: Infection after abdominal surgery: five-year prospective study. Br. med. J. *288:* 278–280 (1984).

5 Condon, R.E.: Prevention of sepsis in treatment of large bowel cancer; in Decosse, Clinical surgery international, vol. 1, large bowel cancer, pp. 63–77 (Churchill, Livingstone 1981).

6 Ljungqvist, U.: Wound sepsis after clean operations. Lancet *i:* 1095–1097 (1964).
7 Bröte, L.: Wound infections in clean and potentially contaminated surgery. Acta chir. scand. *142:* 191–200 (1976).
8 Public Health Laboratory Service. Incidence of surgical wound infection in England and Wales, A Report of the Public Health Laboratory Service. Lancet *ii:* 659–663 (1960).
9 Wenzel, R.P.; Hunting, K.J.; Osterman, C.A.: Postoperative wound infection rates. Surgery Gynec. Obstet. *144:* 749–752 (1977).
10 Strachan, C.: Antibiotic prophylaxis in clean surgical procedures. Wld J. Surg. *6:* 273–280 (1982).
11 Davidson, A.I.G.; Clark, C.; Smith, G.: Postoperative wound infection: a computer analysis. Br. J. Surg. *58:* 333–337 (1971).
12 Cruse, P.J.E.; Foord, R.: A five-year prospective study of 23,649 surgical wounds. Archs Surg., Chicago *107:* 206–210 (1973).
13 Cruse, P.J.E.; Foord, R.: The epidemiology of wound infection: a ten-year prospective study of 62,939 wounds. Surg. Clins N. Am. *60:* 27–40 (1980).
14 Ketcham, A.S.; Lieberman, J.E.; West, J.T.: Antibiotic prophylaxis in cancer surgery and its value in staphylococcal carrier patients. Surgery Gynec. Obstet. *117:* 1–6 (1963).
15 Meakins, J.L. ;Pietsch, J.B.; Christou, N.V.; Maclean, L.V.: Predicting surgical infection before the operation. Wld J. Surg. *4:* 439–450 (1980).
16 Mannell, A.; Plant, M.; Frolich, J.: The microflora of the oesophagus. Ann. R. Coll. Surg. *65:* 152–154 (1983).
17 Lau, W.F.; Wong, J.; Lam, K.H.; Ong, G.B.: Oesophageal microbial flora in carcinoma of oesophagus; in Watts, MacDonald, O'Brien, Marshall, Finlay-Jones, Infection in surgery basic and clinical aspects, pp. 177–180 (Churchill, Livingstone, Edinburgh 1981).
18 Gorbach, S.L.: Intestinal microflora. Gastroenterology *60:* 1110–1129 (1971).
19 Bartlett, J.G.: The normal flora; in Condon, Gorbach, Surgical infections selective antibiotic therapy, pp. 1–6 (Williams & Wilkins, Baltimore 1981).
20 Gorbach, S.L.; Bartlett, J.G.: Anaerobic Infections (first of three parts). New Engl. J. Med. *290:* 1177–1184 (1974).
21 Onderdonk, A.B.; Kasper, D.L.; Cisneros, R.L.; Bartlett, J.G.: The capsular polysaccharide of *Bacteroides fragilis* as a virulence factor: comparison of the pathogenic potential of encapsulated and unencapsulated strains. J. infect. Dis. *136:*82–89 (1977).
22 Ingham, H.R.; Sisson, P.R.; Tharagonnet, D.; Selkon, J.B.; Codd, A.A.: Inhibition of phagocytosis in vitro by obligate anaerobes. Lancet *ii:* 1252–1254 (1977).
23 Brennan, S.S.; Smith, G.M.R.; Evans, M.; Pollock, A.V.: The management of the perforated appendix: a controlled clinical trial. Br. J. Surg. *69:* 510–512 (1982).
24 Tanphiphat, C.; Sangsubhan, C.; Vongvaravipatr, V.: Wound infection in emergency appendicectomy: a prospective trial with topical ampicillin and antiseptic solution irrigation. Br. J. Surg. *65:* 89–91 (1978).
25 Magarey, C.J.; Chant, A.D.B.; Rickford, C.R.K.; Magarey, J.R.: Peritoneal drainage and systemic antibiotics after vasectomy. Lancet *ii:* 179–182 (1971).
26 Pettigrew, R.A.: Delayed primary wound closure in gangrenous and perforated appendicitis. Br. J. Surg. *68:* 635–638 (1981).

27 Foster, G.E.; Bolwell, J.; Balfour, T.W.; Hardcastle, J.D.; Bourke, J.B.; Doran, J.; Holliday, A.; Marshall, D.J.: Clinical and economic consequences of wound sepsis after appendicectomy and then modification by metronidazole or povidone-iodine. Lancet *ii:* 769–771 (1981).

28 Foster, P.D.; O'Toole, R.D.: Primary appendicectomy: the effect of prophylactic cephaloridine on postoperative wound infection. J. Am. med. Ass. *239:* 1411–1412 (1978).

29 Donovan, I.A.; Ellis, D.; Gatehouse, D.; Little, G.; Grimley, R.; Armistead, S.; Keighley, M.R.B.; Strachan, C.J.L.: One-dose antibiotic prophylaxis against wound infection after appendicectomy: a randomised trial of clindomycin, cefazolin sodium and a placebo. Br. J. Surg. *66:* 193–196 (1979).

30 Winslow, R.E.; Dean, R.E.; Harley, J.W.: Acute non-perforating appendicitis: efficacy of brief antibiotic prophylaxis. Archs Surg., Chicago *118:* 651–655 (1983).

31 Hoffman, C.J.; MacDonald, P.J.; Watts, J.M.: Cefoxitin prophylaxis in surgery and non-perforated appendicitis; in Watts, MacDonald, O'Brien, Marshall, Finlay-Jones, Infection in surgery, basic clinical aspects, pp. 217–219 (Churchill, Livingstone 1981).

32 Leigh, D.A.; Pease, R.; Henderson, H.; Simmons, K.; Russ, R.: Prophylactic lincomycin in the prevention of wound infection following appendicectomy: a double-blind study. Br. J. Surg. *63:* 973–977 (1976).

33 Gilmore, O.J.A.; Martin, T.D.M.: Aetiology and prevention of wound infection in appendicectomy. Br. J. Surg. *61:* 281–287 (1974).

34 Pinto, D.J.; Sanderson, P.J.: Rational use of antibiotic therapy after appendicectomy. Br. med. J. *i:* 275–276 (1980).

35 Rogers, J.; Ross, D.; McNaught, W.; Gillespie, G.: Intra-rectal metronidazole in the prevention of anaerobic infections after emergency appendicectomy: a controlled clinical trial. Br. J. Surg. *66:* 425–427 (1979).

36 Kortelainen, P.; Huttunen, R.; Kairaluoma, M.I.; Mokka, R.E.M.; Laitinen, S.; Larmey, T.K.: Single-dose intra-rectal metronidazole prophylaxis against wound infection after appendicectomy. Am. J. Surg. *143:* 244–245 (1982).

37 Greenall, M.J.; Bakran, A.; Pickford, I.R.; Bradley, J.A.; Halsall, A.; McPhie, J.; O'Dell, M.; Cook, E.M.; Lincoln, C.; McMahon, M.J.: A double-blind trial of a single intravenous dose of metronidazole as propyhlaxis against wound infection following appendicectomy. Br. J. Surg. *66:* 428–429 (1979).

38 Longland, C.J.; Gray, J.G.; Pease, W.; Garrett, J.A.M.: The prevention of infection in appendicectomy wounds. Br. J. Surg. *58:* 117–119 (1971).

39 Mountain, J.C.; Seal, P.V.: Topical ampicillin in gridiron appendicectomy wounds. Br. J. clin. Pract. *24:* 111–115 (1970).

40 Bates, T.; Down, R.H.L.; Houghton, M.C.V.; Lloyd, G.J.: Topical ampicillin in the prevention of wound infection after appendicectomy. Br. J. Surg. *61:* 489–492 (1974).

41 Brumer, M.: Appendicitis – Seasonal incidence and postoperative wound infection. Br. J. Surg. *57:* 93–99 (1970).

42 Berne, T.V.; Yellin, A.W.; Appleman, M.D.; Heseltine, P.N.R.: Antibiotic management of surgically treated gangrenous or perforated appendicitis. Am. J. Surg. *144:* 8–13 (1982).

43 Ambrose, N.S.; Donovan, I.A.; Wise, R.; Lowe, P.: Metronidazole and ticarcillin in the prevention of sepsis after appendicectomy. Am. J. Surg. *146:* 346–348 (1983).
44 Morris, W.T.: Control of infection after apendicectomy: metronidazole and cefazolin; in Watts, MacDonald, O'Brien, Marshall, Finlay-Jones, Infection in surgery, basic and clinical aspects, pp. 220–222 (Churchill, Livingstone, Edinburgh 1981).
45 Lau, W.Y.; Fan, S.T.; Yiu, T.F.; Poon, G.P.; Wong, S.H.: Prophylaxis for post-appendicectomy sepsis by metronidazole and cefotaxime: a randomised prospective and double-blind trial. Br. J. Surg. *70:* 670–672 (1983).
46 Andersen, B.; Bentsen, A.; Holbraad, L.; Schantz, A.: Wound infection after appendicectomy. Acta chir. scand. *138:* 531–536 (1972).
47 Rickett, J.W.S.; Jackson, B.T.: Topical ampycillinin the appendicectomy wound. Br. med. J. *iv:* 206–208 (1969).
48 Dupont, P.A.: The efficacy of povidone-iodine (Betadine) in preventing post-appendicectomy wound infections; in Watts, MacDonald, O'Brien, Marshall, Finlay-Jones, Infection in surgery, basic and clinical aspects, pp. 223–226 (Churchill, Livingstone, Edinburgh 1981).
49 Salem, R.J.; Johnson, J.; Devitt, P.: Short-term metronidazole therapy contrasted with povidone-iodine spray in the prevention of wound infection after appendicectomy. Br. J. Surg. *66:* 430–431 (1979).
50 Brooke, I.: Bacterial studies of peritoneal cavity and postoperative surgical wound drainage following perforated appendix in children. Ann. Surg. *192:* 208–212 (1980).
51 Busuttil, R.W.; Davison, R.K.; Fine, M.; Thompkins, K.: Effective prophylactic antibiotics in acute non-perforated appendicitis. Ann. Surg. *194:* 502–509 (1981).
52 Campbell, W.B.: Porphylaxis of infection after appendicectomy: a survey of current surgical practice. Br. med. J. *281:* 1597–1600 (1980).
53 Evans, C.; Pollock, A.V.; Rosenberg, I.L.: The reduction of surgical wound infections by topical cephaloridine: a controlled clinical trial. Br. J. Surg. *61:* 133–135 (1974).
54 Pollock, A.V.; Leaper, D.J.; Evans, M.: Single-dose intra-incisional antibiotic prophyalxis of surgical wound sepsis: a controlled trial of cephaloridine and ampicillin. Br. J. Surg. *64:* 322–325 (1977).
55 Kelly, M.J.; Warren, R.E.: The value of an operative wound swab sent in transport medium in the prediction of later clinical wound infection: a controlled clinical and bacteriological evaluation. Br. J. Surg. *65:* 81–88 (1978).
56 Chodak, G.W.; Plaut, M.E.: Use of systemic antibiotics for prophylaxis in surgery: a critical review. Archs Surg., Chicago *112:* 326–334 (1977).
57 Bartlett, S.P.; Burton, R.C.: Effects of prophylactic antibiotics on wound infection after elective colon and rectal surgery: 1960–1980. Am. J. Surg. *145:* 300–308 (1983).
58 Guglielmo, B.J.; Hohn, D.C.; Koo, P.J.; Hunt, T.K.; Sweet, R.L.; Conte, J.E.: Antibiotic prophylaxis in surgical procedures: a critical analysis of the literature. Archs Surg., Chicago *118:* 943–955 (1983).
59 Giannella, R.A.; Broitman, S.A.; Zamchek, M.: Gastric acid barrier to ingested micro-organisms in man: studies in vivo and in vitro. Gut *13:* 251–256 (1972).
60 Nicholls, R.L.; Smith, J.W.: Intra-gastric microbial colonisation in common disease states of the stomach and duodenum. Ann. Surg. *182:* 557–561 (1975).

61 Gatehouse, D.; Dimock, F.; Burden, D.W.; Alexander-Williams, J.; Keighley, M.R.B.: Prediction of wound sepsis following gastric operations. Br. J. Surg. *65:* 551–554 (1978).
62 Boey, J.; Wong, J.; Ong, G.P.: Bacterial and septic complications in patients with perforated duodenal ulcers. Am. J. Surg. *143:* 635–639 (1982).
63 Nicholls, R.L.; Webb, W.R.; Jones, J.W.; Smith, J.W.; Locicero, J.: Efficacy of antibiotic prophylaxis in high-risk gastroduodenal operations. Am. J. Surg. *143:* 94–98 (1982).
64 Ayres, M.M.; Hegarty, M.A.; Warlow, J.; Mallins, D.; Youngs, D.; Bentley, S.; Burden, D.W.; Keigley, M.R.B.: A control trial to compare systemic and intraincisional cefuroxime prophylaxis in high-risk gastric surgery. Br. J. Surg. *68:* 276–280 (1981).
65 Keighley, M.R.B.: Prevention of wound sepsis in gasto-intestinal surgery. Br. J. Surg. *64:* 315–321 (1977).
66 Lewis, R.T.; Allen, C.M.; Goodall, R.G.; Lloyd-Smith, W.C.; Marian, B.; Wiegand, F.M.: Discriminate use of antibiotic prophylaxis in gastroduodenal surgery. Am. J. Surg. *138:* 640–643 (1979).
67 Gordon-Smith, I.C.; Taylor, E.W.; Nicolaides, A.N.; Golcman, L.; Kenyon, J.R.; Eastcott, H.H.G.: Management of abdominal aortic aneurysm. Br. J. Surg. *65:* 834–838 (1978).
68 Kiser, A.B.; Clayson, K.R.; Mulherin, J.L.; Roach, A.C.; Allen, T.R.; Edwards, W.H.; Dale, W.A.: Antibiotic prophylaxis in vascular surgery. Ann. Surg. *188:* 283–289 (1978).
69 Ernst, C.B.; Campbell, H.C.; Daugherty, M.E.; Sachatello, C.R.; Griffen, W.O.: Incidence and significance of intra-operative bacterial cultures during abdominal aortic aneurysmectomy. Ann. Surg. *185:* 626–633 (1977).
70 Bunt, T.J.: Synthetic vascular graft infections to graft enteric erosions and graft enteric fistulas. Surgery *94:* 1–364 (1983).
71 Wilson, S.E.; Bennion, R.S.; Serota, I.A.; Williams, R.A.: Bacteriological implications in the pathogenesis of secondary aorto-enteric fistulas. Br. J. Surg. *69:* 545–548 (1982).
72 Pitt, A.J.; Postier, R.G.; MacGowan, W.L.; Frank, L.W.; Sermack, A.J.; Sitzman, J.V.; Bouchier-Hayes, D.: Prophylactic antibiotics in vascular surgery: topical systemic or both? Ann. Surg. *192:* 356–364 (1980).
73 Sellwood, R.A.; Burren, J.I.; Waterwork, P.M.; Welbourne, R.B.: A second clinical trial to compare two methods for pre-operative preparation of the large bowel. Br. J. Surg. *56:* 610–612 (1969).
74 Nicholls, R.L.; Broido, P.; Condon, R.E.; Gorbach, S.L.; Nyhus, L.M.: Effective pre-operative neomycin erythromycin intestinal preparation on the incidence of infectious complications following colon surgery. Ann. Surg. *178:* 453–461 (1973).
75 Clark, J.S.; Condon, R.E.; Bartlett, J.G.; Gorbach, S.L.; Nicholls, R.L.; Ochi, S.: Pre-operative oral antibiotics reduce septic complications of colon operations: results of prospective, randomised, double-blind clinical study. Ann. Surg. *186:* 251–259 (1977).
76 Bartlett, J.G.; Condon, R.E.; Gorbach, S.L.; Clark, J.S.; Nicholls, R.L.; Ochi, S.: Veteran's Administration Cooperative Study on Bowel Preparation for Elective Colo-

Rectal Operations: impact of oral antibiotic regimen on colonic flora and irrigation cultures and bacteriology of septic complications. Ann. Surg. *188:* 249–254 (1978).

77 Washington, J.A.; Dearing, W.H.; Judd, E.S.; Elvibach, L.R.: Effective preoperative antibiotic regimen on development of infection after intestinal surgery: prospective randomised double-blind study. Ann. Surg. *180:* 567–572 (1974).

78 Goldring, J.; McNaught, W.; Scott, A.; Gillespie, G.: Prophylactic oral antimicrobial agents in elective colonic surgery: a controlled trial. Lancet *ii:* 997–999 (1975).

79 Matheson, D.M.; Arabi, Y.; Baxter-Smith, D.; Alexander-Williams, J.; Keighley, M.R.B.: Randomised, multi-centre trial of oral bowel preparation and antimicrobials for elective colo-rectal operations. Br. J. Surg. *65:* 597–600 (1978).

80 Arabi, Y.; Dimock, F.; Burden, D.W.; Alexander-Williams, J.; Keighley, M.R.B.: Influence of noemycin and metronidazole on colonic microflora of volunteers. J. antimicrob. Chemother. *5:* 531–537 (1979).

81 Wapnik, S.; Guintor-Reizis, I.; Leveen, H.H.: Reduction of postoperative infection in elective colon surgery with pre-operative administration of kanamycin and erythromycin. Surgery *85:* 317–321 (1979).

82 Polk, H.C.; Lopez-Mayor, J.F.: Postoperative wound infection: a prospective study of determinant factors and prevention. Surgery *66:* 97–103 (1969).

83 Stone, H.H.; Hooper, C.A.; Colb, L.D.; Geheber, C.E.; Dorkins, E.J.: Antibiotic prophylaxis in gastric, biliary and colonic surgery. Ann. Surg. *184:* 443–452 (1976).

84 Feathers, R.S.; Lewis, A.A.M.; Sagor, G.R.; Amirak, I.D.; Noon, P.: Prophylactic systemic antibiotics in colo-rectal surgery. Lancet *ii:* 4–8 (1977).

85 Willis, A.T.; Ferguson, I.R.; Jones, P.H.; Phillips, K.D.; Tearle, P.V.; Fiddian, R.V.; et al.: Metronidazole in prevention and treatment of Bacteroides infections in elective colonic surgery. Br. med. J. *i:* 607–610 (1977).

86 Hoffman, C.E.; MacDonald, H.A.; Watts, J.M.: Short-course prophylaxis with cefoxitin in colo-rectal surgery; in Watts, MacDonald, O'Brien, Marshall, Finlay-Jones, Infection in surgery, basic and clinical aspects, pp. 260–263 (Churchill, Livingstone, Edinburgh 1981).

87 Keighley, M.R.B.; Crapp, A.R.; Burden, D.W.; Cook, W.T.; Alexander-Williams, J.: Prophylaxis against anaerobic sepsis in bowel surgery. Br. J. Surg. *63:* 538–541 (1976).

88 Hojer, H.; Wetterfors, J.: Systemic prophylaxis with doxycycline in surgery of the colon and rectum. Ann. Surg. *187:* 362–368 (1978).

89 Bjerkeset, T.; Digranes, A.: Systemic prophylaxis with metronidazole (Flagyl) in effective surgery of the colon and rectum. Surgery *87:* 560–565 (1980).

90 Mittermayer, H.; Gross, C.; Brucke, P.: Prophylaxis with single-dose cefuroxime/metronidazole versus metronidazole alone in elective colo-rectal surgery. Res. clin. Forums *5:* 109–119 (1982).

91 Mitchell, M.J.; Evans, D.S.; Pollock, D.: Single-dose metronidazole with and without cefuroxime in elective colorectal surgery. Br. J. Surg. *70:* 668–669 (1983).

92 Morris, D.L.; Hares, M.M.; Voogt, R.J.; Burden, J.W.; Keighley, M.R.B.: Metronidazole need not be combined with an aminoglycoside when used for prophylaxis in elective colorectal surgery. J. Hosp. Infect. *4:* 65–69 (1983).

93 Keighley, M.R.B.; Arabi, Y.; Alexander-Williams, J.; Youngs, D.; Burden, D.W.: Comparison between systemic and oral antimicrobial prophylaxis in colorectal surgery. Lancet *ii:* 894–897 (1979).

94 Hansell, D.T.; Thompson, D.J.L.; Simpson, C.J.; Moran, C.; Smith, D.C.; MacNaughton, W.; Gillespie, G.: Metronidazole prophylaxis in colorectal surgery: the need for additional aminoglycoside J. Hosp. Infect. *4:* 383–390 (1983).
95 Dion, Y.M.; Richards, G.K.; Prentice, J.J.; Hinchey, J.: The influence of oral versus parenteral pre-operative metronidazole on sepsis following colon surgery. Ann. Surg. *192:* 221–226 (1980).
96 Eykyn, S.J.; Jackson, B.T.; Lockhart-Mummery, A.G.; Phillips, I.: Prophylactic peri-operative intravenous metronidazole in elective colorectal surgery. Lancet *ii:* 761–764 (1979).
97 Taylor, S.A.; Cawdrey, H.M.; Smith, J.: The use of metronidazole in the preparation of the bowel for surgery. Br. J. Surg. *66:* 191–192 (1979).
98 Higgins, A.F.; Lewis, A.; Noon, P.; Hole, M.L.: Single- and multiple-dose cotrimoxazole and metronidazole in colorectal surgery. Br. J. Surg. *67:* 90–92 (1980).
99 Brown, J.J.; Mutton, T.P.; Wasilauskas, B.L.; Myers, R.T.; Meredith, J.H.: Prospective randomised control trial of ticazillin and cefalothin as prophylactic antibiotics for gastro-intestinal operations. Am. J. Surg. *143:* 343–348 (1982).
100 Ivarson, L.; Darrell, N.; Kewenter, J.G.; Seeberg, S.; Norrby, R.: Short-term systemic prophylaxis with cefoxitin and doxycycline in colorectal surgery: a prospective randomised study. Am. J. Surg. *144:* 257–261 (1982).
101 Stamatakis, J.D.; Binu, P.S.; Strachan, C.J.L.: Prevention of wound and intra-abdominal sepsis following left colorectal resection. Coloproc. *4:* 222–225 (1982).
102 Coppa, G.F.; Eng, K.; Gouge, T.H.; Ranson, J.H.; Localio, S.A.: Parenteral and oral antibiotics inelective colon and rectal surgery. Am. J. Surg. *145:* 60–65 (1983).
103 Stewart, M.; Failes, D.; Kellingbach, M.J.: Wound infection in elective colorectal surgery – A prospective study with kanamycin and metronidazole; in Watts, MacDonald, O'Brien, Marshall, Finlay-Jones, Infection in surgery, basic and clinical aspects, pp. 264–265 (Churchill, Livingstone, Edinburgh 1981).
104 Condon, R.E.: Bowel preparation for colorectal operations. Archs Surg., Chicago *117:* 265 (1982).
105 Wilson, N.I.L.; Wright, P.A.; MacCardal, C.S.: Survey of antibiotic prophylaxis in gastro-intestinal surgery in Scotland. Br. med. J. *285:* 871–873 (1982).
106 MacDonald, P.J.; Karran, S.J.: Pre-operative antimicrobial prescribing practice for elective colorectal surgery in Wessex 1981. Lancet *ii:* 753–754 (1982).
107 Ambrose, N.S.; Burden, D.W.; Keighley, M.R.B.: Prospective randomised trial to compare mezlocillin and metronidazole with cefuroxime and metronidazole as prophylaxis in elective colorectal operations. J. Hosp. Infect. *4:* 375–382 (1983).
108 Baum, M.L.; Annisch, D.S.; Chalmers, T.C.; Sacks, H.S.; Smith, H.; Fagarstrom, R.M.: A survey of clinical trials of antibiotic prophylaxis in colon surgery: evidence against further use of no-treatment controls. New Engl. J. Med. *305:* 795–799 (1981).
109 Arabi, Y.; Dimock, F.; Burden, D.W.; Alexander-Williams, J.; Keighley, M.R.B.: Influence of bowel preparation and antimicrobials, colonic microflora. Br. J. Surg. *65:* 555–559 (1978).
110 Nicholls, R.L.; Gorbach, R.L.; Condon, R.E.: Alteration of intestinal microflora following pre-operative mechanical preparation of the colon. Dis. Col. Rect. *14:* 123–127 (1971).

111 Wise, R.: A review of the antimicrobial and pharmacological properties of the penicillins and cephalosporins. Res. clin. Forums *5:* 1-13 (1983).
112 National Academy of Sciences - National Research Council, Division of Medical Sciences: Postoperative wound infections, the influence of ultraviolet irradiation of the operating room and various other factors. Ann. Surg. *160:* suppl. 1 (1964).
113 Beatty, D.J.; Robinson, G.V.; Zaia, J.A.; Benfield, J.R.; Kemery, M.; Meguid, M.M.; Riihimaki, D.U.; Terz, J.J.; Lemmelin, M.E.: A prospective analysis of nosocomial wound infection after mastectomy. Archs Surg., Chicago *118:* 1421-1424 (1983).

A.J. Wilson, MSC, MD, FRCS(G), 11 Tulsemere Rd., West Norwood, London SE27 (UK)

Antibiot. Chemother., vol. 33, pp. 59–72 (Karger, Basel 1985)

Prevention of Infection in High Risk Biliary Operations

S.J. Karran, M. de la Hunt, I. Townend, G. Tasker, B. Walmsley, P. McDonald, C. Royce, H. Goh, R. Dawes, J. Smallwood, J. Browning, S. Scott, A.J. Papachristodoulou, G. Sutton, P. Reddy, V. O'Malley

University Surgical Unit, Faculty of Medicine, Southampton General Hospital, Southampton, UK

Every operation is an exercise in bacteriology [1]. The fact that the degree of risk varies widely has been acknowledged for many years but controversy remains over many aspects of postoperative sepsis. In this review an attempt will be made to discuss critically the importance of several factors which influence clinical outcome. No apology is made for personal conclusions and beliefs.

Essential to the debate must be an appreciation of the multifactorial nature of the problem. It is clear that not only 'local' factors, related to the pathology of the biliary tree and its surgery (table I, II), but also 'general' (i.e. host) and 'environmental' factors are important in the development of postoperative septic complications (fig. 1).

In addition, the distinction between incidence and consequence of postoperative sepsis must be emphasised. The frequent occurrence of minor septic complications obviously has a different significance from infrequent but life threatening sepsis. Prophylactic measures are thus of importance not only to reduce the frequency of septic complications, but are justified to prevent loss of life even when the incidence is low. Open heart and hip replacement procedures are obvious examples where antibiotic therapy is justified for this reason. The complex relationship between true prophylaxis and treatment of established sepsis is summarised in fig. 2.

Which Patients Are at Risk Undergoing Biliary Surgery?

In recent years there have been several studies which have clearly demonstrated factors associated with an increased risk of postopera-

Table I. Surgeon-related factors

1	Contamination, e.g. bile, feces
2	Hematoma
3	Tissue damage
4	Ischemia
5	Slowness – unnecessary exposure to environment
6	Foreign materials, particularly braided sutures
7	Poor discipline, e.g. movement, visitors, talking, masks, carriers

Table II. Approximate risk of septic complications, e.g. wound sepsis, that may be expected in different areas of surgical practice, without the use of antibiotics, according to the technical expertise of the surgeon

Type of surgery	Sepsis rate according to degree of surgical expertise, %		
	high	average	poor
Clean			
Hernias, varicose veins, breast surgery, orthopedics, vascular surgery	0.2	2	5
Potentially contaminated			
Low risk, Biliary, gastric surgery	3	10	20
High risk, Colorectal surgery (elective)	15	45	70
Contaminated			
Peritonitis, drainage of abscesses	75	85	100

tive wound sepsis (table III) [2–4]. There is little debate about the relevance of these factors, but other issues remain contentious.

Audit and Pathology

It is difficult to determine the incidence of high risk factors in the clinical practice of certain surgeons, especially those who claim that they 'see no sepsis'. It has ever been true that there are 'none so blind as will not see'. Only when accurate prospective audit is performed can valid assessment be made. Polk has aptly described the retrospectivists as expert practitioners of the art of 'selective forgetfulness'. In Wessex since 1975 we have conducted several prospective studies of antimic-

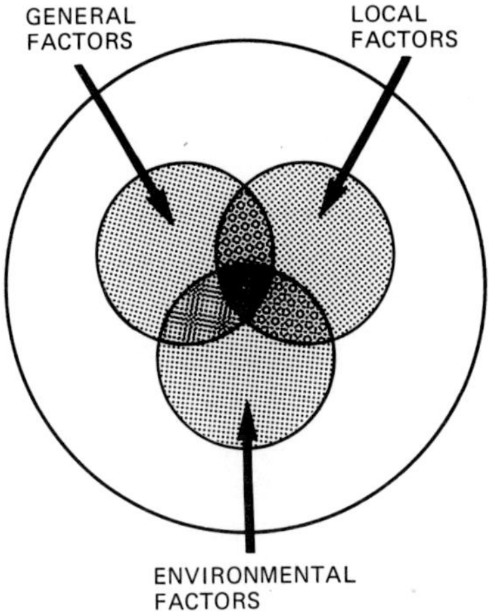

Fig. 1. Interrelationship between local, general and environmental factors in the production of sepsis.

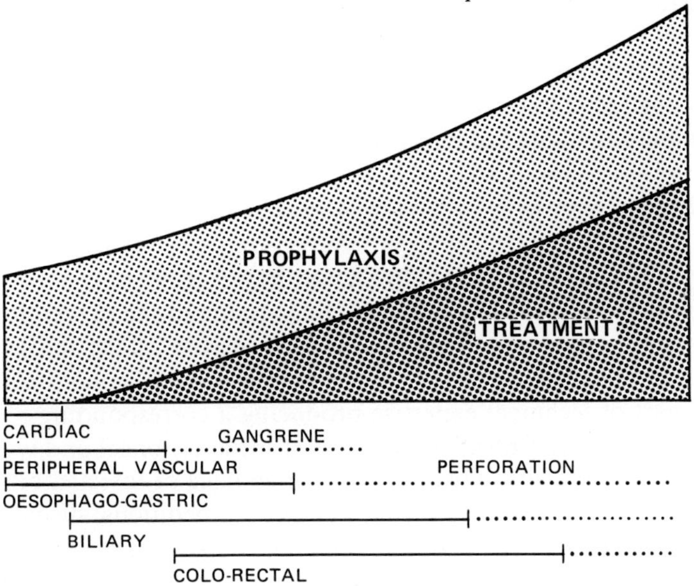

Fig. 2. Complex relationship between prophylaxis and treatment of established sepsis.

robial prophylaxis in elective biliary surgery in well over 1,000 patients. In these studies there has been at least one high risk factor identifiable in over 60% of patients. In a further 10% two or more factors have been found [unpublished data]. Whilst this may be a criticism of the British National Health Service, it is clear that such a pattern of

Table III. High risk factors in biliary surgery

1	Emergency surgery
2	Age > 70
3	Jaundice
4	Obesity
5	Exploration of common bile duct
6	Concomitant alimentary procedures, e.g. appendicectomy, biliary by-pass
7	Previous biliary surgery
8	Malnutrition
9	Immunosuppression
10	Diabetes

surgical practice is not identical in all parts of the world. Indeed, it has been stated in certain communities that the incidence of cholecystectomies performed is proportional not to the prevalence of cholelithiasis, but rather to the number of surgeons in town! It takes little insight to appreciate that surgeons consistently operating on minimal pathology, with its negligible bacterial load, should have wound infection rates comparable with those for herniorrhaphies.

Surgical Expertise

With differences in pathology apart, however, there is absolutely no doubt that the most important single variable in the prevention of postoperative septic complications is the expertise of the individual surgeon. Immaculate attention to prevention of contamination is an integral part of technical expertise producing a corresponding reduction in postoperative infection. The use of intraperitoneal and wound protectors, and the absolute avoidance of spillage of infected bile are but two obvious examples of this expertise. Expeditious, disciplined and delicate surgery, through the reduction of exogenous contamination, is also of obvious merit. Some of these major surgeon-related variables are summarised in table I. In Great Britain at least 50% of elective biliary procedures are performed by surgeons in training, whilst in other countries it is probable that a higher proportion is undertaken by independent practitioners. This may have some bearing on differences in reported sepsis rates.

Possible explanations for the widely differing reports of postoperative sepsis rates thus include variations in accuracy of audit, severity of underlying pathology and individual surgical expertise.

Patient Selection for Chemoprophylaxis

In an ideal world surgical procedures would be performed without the need for adjuvant antimicrobial therapy. As already emphasised, with meticulous attention to proven principles of asepsis and other aspects of surgical technique, postoperative septic complications should be reduced to a minimum. It is generally agreed that wound sepsis rates of greater than 2% for 'clean' cases are not acceptable [5, 6]. No reliable prospective studies have yet been performed to show that this can be achieved in elective biliary surgery without the use of antimicrobial agents. Whilst it is generally agreed that all high risk cases described in table III are worthy of antibiotic 'protection', there has been reluctance to provide prophylactic therapy for other patients undergoing elective biliary surgery. The suggestion has been made that microscopic examination of bile obtained at operation may be of value in selecting additional patients for antibiotic therapy. This suggestion has never commended itself to us as it is illogical. The technique takes at least 20 min to perform even in expert hands, so that by the time the result is known the patient will have been 'at risk' for probably double that period, depending on the speed with which the bile has been collected for examination. Administration of an antibiotic at this delayed juncture thus contravenes the basic and now firmly established principle of prophylaxis, which is that clean uninfected tissues (e.g. the wound) should be 'loaded' with the appropriate antibiotic immediately before the period of risk.

A second disadvantage of this technique is that over 30% of organisms present may be missed [7] and the final condemnation of this approach is in the results of two prospective studies from Manchester [7] and Glasgow [8) which showed that patients selected by the method (even when considerable experience into the technique had been obtained) fared no better than untreated controls!

Which Antibiotics and by Which Route?

Criteria for choosing an appropriate antimicrobial agent are clearly defined. It must obviously possess an appropriate spectrum of activity against those organisms likely to be responsible for septic complications. The risk of bacterial contamination is not only from exogenous but, more particularly, from endogenous sources. A schematic representation of this risk is shown in figure 3. Whilst staphylococci constitute the major hazard from exogenous contamination, the organisms causing endogenous contamination comprise the enteric bacteria shown in table IV. Although anaerobic organisms are occasionally implicated [9], particularly in the elderly or in patients with parasitic infestation [10], these do not normally constitute a significant hazard in elective biliary surgery. Indeed, in a prospective study [11] it was shown that prophylactic administration of metronidazole offered no advantage compared with the placebo control group.

Perusal of manufacturers' literature soon makes it apparent that there is an abundance, in fact a superfluity, of antibiotics which exhibit potent activity against these organisms. Choice of an agent for prophylaxis should then be made on the basis of objective clinical trial data, pharmacokinetic information and, ultimately, cost. Of the many antibiotics evaluated in recent years most have been β-lactam compounds, principally the cephalosporins.

Our own prospective studies in the Wessex region of Britain commenced in 1975. These were the first studies undertaken evaluating *single-dose* prophylaxis and over the years many other centres, particularly Birmingham [12], Frimley Park [13], Glasgow [8] and Manchester [7] have also adopted this approach. Although methods such as intramuscular injection and intra-incisional instillation of antibiotic [14] have been used [15], the intravenous route of administration, infusing the antibiotic over a period of a few minutes commencing immediately the patient is hemodynamically stable after induction of anesthesia, is now firmly established as the method of choice. Many centers in the United States, however, have yet to adopt this logical approach still preferring the intramuscular route at the time of premedication. In the rare event that an anaphylactic reaction should occur, if the patient is already intubated and in the care of a competent anesthetist no harm should befall. In 9 years of the use of single-dose antibiotic prophylaxis in Southampton we have yet to meet this complication, as all patients with potential antibiotic hypersensitivity have been excluded from our studies. When a high risk patient with a probable hypersensitivity to penicillin is encountered, a single 120 mg prophylactic dose of gentamicin is employed. This would appear to be one of the rare occasions when an aminoglycoside is justified for prophylaxis.

In the first of our prospective studies undertaken in 1975 we compared a group of patients given a 2 gram intramuscular dose of the ce-

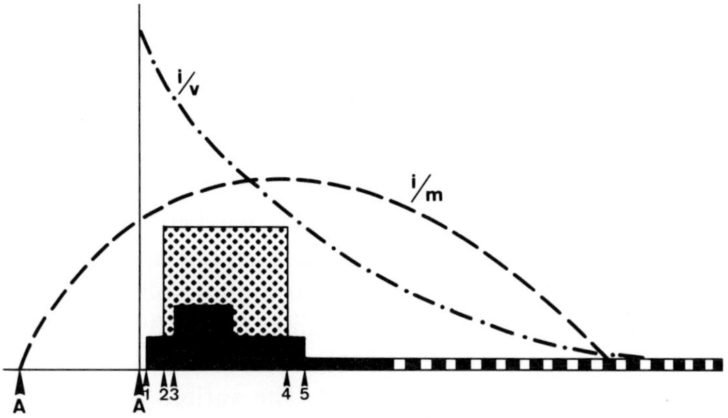

Fig. 3. Period of risk of contamination in biliary surgery. 1 = Initial incision - start of exogenous risk; 2 = dissection of gallbladder and biliary tree - start of period of endogenous risk; 3 = peroperative radiology with increased risk of exogenous contamination; 4 = ligation of cystic duct marking end of period of potential endogenous risk; 5 = closure of wound - end of major component of exogenous risk, followed by wound healing. Exogenous risk means especially by gram-positive cocci; and endogenous risk means especially *E. coli, Klebsiella, S. faecalis.* i/m = Serum and tissue levels produced by single dose intramuscular antibiotic administration at time of premedication; i/v = levels produced by intravenous administration at time of induction of anesthesia.

*Fig. 4.*Serum level profiles in intra-venous administration.

Table IV. Bacteria most commonly found in the biliary tree (198 positive cultures) [20]

Gram-negative		
Escherichia coli	67	
Klebsiella aerogenes	32	
Mixed coliforms	27	
Pseudomonas spp.	9	
	135	(69%)
Gram-positive		
Enterococci	22	
Streptococci	18	
Staphylococci	11	
Diphteroids	7	
Bacteroides spp.	2	
Clostridium spp.	3	
	63	(31%)

phalosporin cephazolin with an untreated group of patients [4]. A 10% reduction in wound sepsis prompted institution of a full double-blind study comparing this therapy with a 2-gram dose of placebo (the placebo was not available at the time of the initial study). Similar benefit was shown in this second study (table V).

In 1977 considerable controversy existed over the importance of the protein binding (PB) of an antibiotic [15]. We therefore undertook a study to compare the clinical value of three cephalosporins of widely differing protein binding, but with similar antimicrobial activity [16]. The antibiotics studied were cephradine (PB ≙ 10%), cefuroxime (PB ≙ 30%) and cefamandole (PB ≙ 80%). A placebo group was also included in this study (for the last time!). The antibiotics and placebo were administered intravenously immediately after induction of anesthesia and serum levels achieved are shown in figure 4 for both free and bound compounds.

In the placebo group wound infections occurred in 4 out of 25 patients (16%), compared with none of the antibiotic-treated patients. There was, in addition, a 30% reduction in proven respiratory tract and other postoperative infections in these treated patients compared with the placebo control patients. It appeared that there was little to choose between the different antibiotics studied, despite wide differences in protein binding, particularly so far as wound infection was concerned. Also, as a result of this study it was deemed unethical to use a no-treatment group in our subsequent studies.

In subsequent usage cephazolin was shown to be associated with a less than 1% wound infection rate in elective biliary surgery (n = 125) when 2 g were administered intravenously after induction as described.

In recent years a veritable plethora of new antibiotics has been introduced into clinical practice. Many of these compounds, principally second and third generation cephalosporins, have been advocated vociferously by the manufacturers for infections of the biliary tract. Whilst these compounds are attractive on the basis of in vitro activity, their precise role in surgical practice is less clear. This is especially true when the manufacturers have not deigned to submit them to carefully designed and performed prospective clinical trials, but have relied instead on other methods of advocacy! We have therefore undertaken a series of prospective comparative trials within the Wessex region over the last 7 years to try to elucidate the place of many of these compounds. To date, the following antibiotics have been studied, in addi-

Table V. High risk factors in 2 initial studies (from ref. 4, with permission)

	Cephazolin	Control
Number of patients	24	25
Number over 60 years	10	10
Number over 70 kg	9	6
Jaundice (bilirubin > 20 μmol/l, [1.2 mg/dl])	4	6
Biliary tree explored	1	5
Emergency surgery	4	–
Concomitant alimentary[1] surgery	9	9
Total risk factors	37	36
Number/patient	1.54	1.44
	Control	**Cephazolin**
Number of patients	48[2]	49[2]
Age > 70 years	6 (12.2%)	6 (12.5%)
Weight > 70 kg	11 (25%)	11 (25%)
Jaundice	9 (18%)	6 (13%)
Biliary tree explored	2	6
Emergency surgery	–	–
Concomitant alimentary surgery	5	3
Total	33	32
Risk factor per patient	0.68	0.65

[1] Appendicectomy, choledochojejunostomy, etc.
[2] Patients withdrawn from trial because of incorrect preoperative diagnosis and non-biliary pathology discovered at laparotomy.

tion to those already mentioned above: mezlocillin (n = 75), piperacillin (n = 30), cefoxitin (n = 75), ceftriaxone (n = 90), timentin (n = 50) and claforan (n = 70).

With regard to wound infections, no significant difference between antibiotics has been seen. Indeed, it is clear that several thousands of patients would be required in any study to demonstrate statistically significant differences. Differences between any of these excellent antibiotics and placebo, however, are easily demonstrated. In our

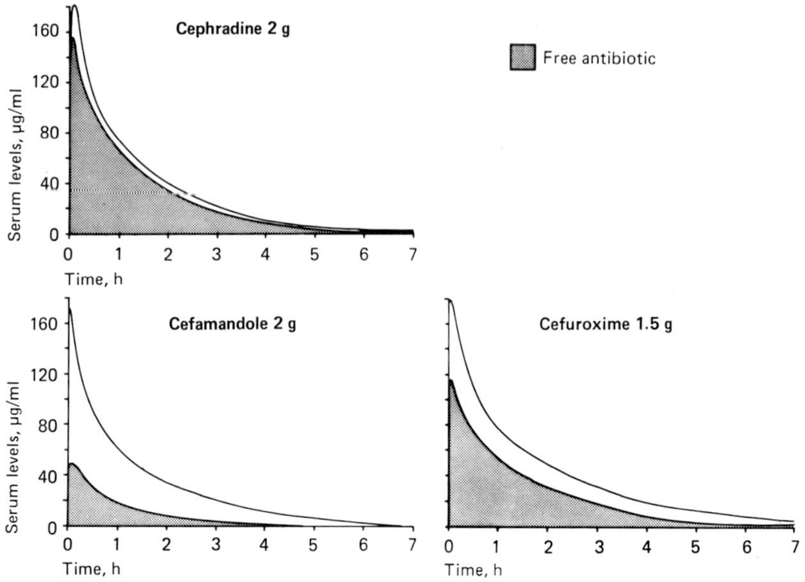

Fig. 4. Serum level profiles intra-venous administration.

experience a single i.v. 2-gram dose of any of the compounds studied is associated with a less than 1% in-hospital wound sepsis rate. However, an additional 2% late infection rate occurs within 1 month of discharge from hospital. When surgical misdemeanours such as biliary (or enteric) leakage or hematoma formation occur, sepsis rates will inevitably be increased. It is irrational to hope that a short course of antibiotic prophylaxis (of approximately 4 h duration) can obscure fundamental surgical errors. The fact that antibiotic therapy can hide surgical evils of lesser magnitude, however, has been a potent hindrance to our advocacy of this proven adjuvant approach to patient care. The concern of all surgeons should rightly be to achieve the highest possible standards of surgical expertise. Although antibiotics will never convert a third rate surgeon into a master of the craft, failure by the latter to utilise this rational therapy in his practice must surely relegate him to the lower divisions! The onus now is clearly on surgeons who refuse to admit the merit of short course prophylaxis, to prove in a large scale, properly audited, prospective study, that they can achieve equal benefit for their patients by avoiding prophylaxis!

Another facet of considerable interest and controversy is the incidence, and indeed severity, of postoperative respiratory infections in biliary surgery. Although evidence has been slower to accumulate, it is my conviction that additional benefits are to be gained in this area, even with the use of single dose prophylaxis [17, 18]. As already mentioned, in one of our early studies [16] we observed a 3-fold reduction in chest infections (proven by established radiological and/or bacteriological criteria) in antibiotic-treated patients compared with untreated patients. Similar results have since been reported in two other prospective studies [17, 18]. In our own later studies it has not been possible on ethical grounds to repeat our early observation, as all our patients have received antibiotic prophylaxis because of the proven benefit in wound sepsis prevention. When treated patients, however, are compared with similar patients not included in these studies, a similar difference has been observed in the incidence of clinical chest infections. In addition, in an analysis of the postoperative temperature charts of these two groups of patients, the area 'under the curve' is very greatly reduced in antibiotic-treated patients. Whilst this does not, in itself, prove that this benefit is solely due to the effect of the antibiotics on the respiratory tract, it is further corroborative evidence.

A more surprising observation that we have made in a recent study has been a highly significant difference between two antibiotics. The new cephalosporin, ceftriaxone (Rocephin) is of particular interest because of its extremely protracted half-life (approximately 6 h). This antibiotic has recently been compared with cephradine (at present one of the most widely used cephalosporins in the UK) in a prospective study of 140 patients undergoing elective biliary surgery [19]. The half-life of ceftriaxone is approximately 4 times greater than that of cephradine, and although there was no difference in the incidence of wound infections in either group of patients, the incidence of either proven chest infections, suspected chest infections, or occasions when the clinician subsequently prescribed a course of antibiotics, was 3 times lower in the ceftriaxone group ($p < 0.001$). In the early postanesthetic period when secretions cannot readily be cleared from the bronchial tree because of increased viscosity, and when patients' ventilatory efforts are reduced by the pain from an upper abdominal incision, the scene is clearly set for respiratory infection. A single 2-gram dose of ceftriaxone gives at least a 12-hour antibacterial 'cover' and this is the probable reason for its beneficial effect. Further studies to evaluate this observation are proceeding.

Economics of Chemoprophylaxis

In the present climate of financial stringency the easily identifiable high cost of antimicrobials in the hospital budget is of universal concern. In addition, when it is seen that by far the greatest proportion of antibiotic prescribing in surgery in many centers is for prophylaxis, it is hardly surprising that questions are asked by administrators. It is not perhaps surprising, however, that certain conclusions currently drawn from such examination of expenditure are not only irrational, but also potentially dangerous.

Whilst no right-minded administrator would question the use of clinically beneficial therapy, certain illogical arguments are not always refuted as they should be. In particular, the economic facts pertinent to rational chemoprophylaxis must be carefully considered. Clearly no clinician can defend the use of an expensive therapy which carries little benefit. On occasions, however, clinicians lay themselves open to criticism by yielding to the temptation to use a new 'wonder' drug, whether this be for excitement, fashion, or worse.

What then is the economic position for elective biliary surgery? As already pointed out, in the UK the majority of patients (≙70%) are at an increased risk of developing postoperative septic complications. As we have demonstrated consistently over the last 8 years, these complications can be virtually eliminated by the judicious use of single-dose chemoprophylaxis. The magnitude of this reduction in wound sepsis is at least 5%, and probably nearer 10% in most hospitals. Serious wound infections delay discharge from hospital by 2–3 days, resulting in a wastage of at least 10–30 patient days for every 100 'unprotected' patients undergoing elective biliary surgery. At present in the UK, the hospital cost for surgical patients is approximately £100 per day. Most of this is 'hotel' (>30%) and nursing cost (>20%), thus between £1,000 and £3,000 are wasted as a result of avoidable septic complications when chemoprophylaxis is not employed. The cost of prescribing 2 g of cephazolin, on the other hand, to all 100 patients is approximately £600!

Unfortunately, it is not usually possible to extend the argument into a positive one of saving money through rational use of chemoprophylaxis, because greater efficiency in patient management by surgeons is, with increasing frequency, met by a reduction in the number of hospital beds and operating time, and withdrawal of nursing services by too many administrators.

The least that any clinician can do in these circumstances, however, is to prove the clinical value of carefully considered policies through rigorous prospective audit. He may thus best resist the unholy clamor of ill-informed pressure groups, who are so blinkered that they can see only their own budgetary corner rather than the vista of total patient management.

Dangers of Prophylaxis

At the end of the day each surgeon must weigh up for himself the evidence for and against prophylaxis in each individual patient. Although, in our opinion, the scales are tipped heavily in favor of single-dose prophylaxis for virtually all patients undergoing elective biliary surgery, constant vigilance is essential for potential hazards. If extremely potent long-acting antimicrobials, such as ceftriaxone, become widely used, there is danger of some patients developing life-threatening pseudomembranous colitis, particularly if these agents are excreted well in bile [*Lacey,* personal commun.]. Other hazards of induced resistance and toxic or hypersensitivity reactions are also very real. We have not, however, experienced these problems in our prospective studies carried out over this 9-year period, as patients with possible hypersensitivity to β-lactam antibiotics have been excluded from the studies. Despite potential risks it is our firm contention that rational single-dose chemoprophylaxis in virtually all patients undergoing elective biliary surgery is not only simple and safe, but is of proven clinical benefit. It also makes economic sense.

References

1 Moynihan: The ritual of a surgical operation. 1st meet. Ass. Surgeons, London 1920.
2 Chetlin, S.H.; Elliott, D.W.: Biliary bacteraemia. Archs Surg. *102:* 303–307 (1971).
3 Keighley, M.R.B.; Flinn, R.; Alexander-Williams, J.: Multivariate analysis of clinical and operative findings associated with biliary sepsis. Br. J. Surg. *63:* 528–531 (1976).

4 Papachristodoulou, A.J.; Mackenzie, A.; Norman, J.; Karran, S.J.: Single dose cephazolin prophylaxis in biliary tract surgery. J. R. Coll. Surg., Edinburgh *23:* 178–183 (1978).
5 Cruse, P.J.E.: Surgical infection surveillance; in Karran, Controversies in surgical sepsis, chapt. 27, pp. 327–322 (Praeger, New York 1980).
6 Birnbaum, D.: Risk management versus infection control committees. Dimensions *58:* 16–19 (1981).
7 Gallagher, P.; Ostick, G.; Jones, D.; Schofield, P.F.; Tweedle, D.E.F.: Intra-operative microscopy of bile – is it useful? Br. J. Surg. *69:* 473–474 (1982).
8 Murray, W.R.; Bradley, J.A.: Antibiotic prophylaxis in elective biliary surgery. Res. clin. Forums *5:* 97–102 (1983).
9 Keighley, M.R.B.: Microorganisms in the bile. A preventable cause of sepsis after biliary surgery. Ann. R. Coll. Surg. *59:* 328–334 (1977).
10 Shimada, K.; Inamatsu, T.; Yamashiro, M.: Anaerobic bacteria in biliary disease in elderly patients. J. infect. dis. *135:* 850–854 (1977).
11 Halsall, A.K.; Welsh, C.L.; Craven, J.L.; Hopton, D.S.; Peel, R.N.: Prophylactic use of metronidazole in preventing wound sepsis after elective cholecystectomy. Br. J. Surg. *67:* 551–552 (1980).
12 Strachan, C.J.L.; Black, J.; Powis, S.J.A.; Waterworth, T.A.; Wise, R.; Wilkinson, A.R.; Burdon, D.W.; Severn, M.; Mitra, B.; Norcott, H.: Prophylactic use of cephazolin against wound sepsis after cholecystectomy. Br. med. J. *i:* 1254–1256 (1977).
13 Batch, A.J.G.; Amery, A.H.; Lallemand, R.C.: Prophylactic cephazolin in biliary surgery. Proc. 5th Wld Gastro-enterology Congr., Sao Paulo 1978.
14 Taylor, T.V.; Walker, W.S.; Mason, R.C.; Richmond, J.; Lee, D.: Preoperative intraparietal (intra incisional) cefoxitin in abdominal surgery. Br. J. Surg. *69:* 461–462 (1982).
15 Selwyn, S.: Discussion on chemoprophylaxis; in Karran, Controversies in surgical sepsis, pp. 172–173 (Praeger, New York 1980).
16 Karran, S.J.; Lewington, V.; Allen, S.; Cooper, A.; McDonald, P.J.: Prospective double blind evaluation of single dose intravenous prophylaxis using three cephalosporins in biliary surgery. Proc. XVI Congr. Eur. Soc. Surg. Res., Garmisch-Partenkirchen 1981 (Karger, Basel 1981).
17 Morran, C.; McNaught, W.; McArdle, C.S.: Prophylactic cotrimoxazole in biliary surgery. Br. med. J. *ii:* 462–464 (1978).
18 McArdle, C.S.; Morran, C.G.; Thomson, S.; White, A.; Pickard, R.; McNaught, W.; Smith, D.C.: Prophylactic cefuroxime in biliary surgery. Res. clin. Forums *5:* 65–72 (1983).
19 Hunt, M.H. de la; Karran, S.J.: A comparison of the long acting cephalosporin, ceftriaxone, with cephradine for prophylaxis of elective biliary surgery. Proc. 4th Med. Cong. Chemother., Rhodes, Greece, October 1984 (in press).
20 Elliott, D.W.: Prevention of sepsis in biliary surgery; in Karran, Controversies in surgical sepsis, p. 286 (Praeger, New York).

S.J. Karran, MChir, F.R.C.S., FRCS Ed., University Surgical Unit,
Faculty of Medicine, Southampton General Hospital,
Tremona Road, Southampton, S01 6HU (UK)

Antibiot. Chemother., vol. 33, pp. 73–89 (Karger, Basel 1985)

Perioperative Antibiotics for Hysterectomy

David L. Hemsell

Department of Obstetrics and Gynecology, University of Texas Health Science Center at Dallas, Southwestern Medical School, Parkland Memorial Hospital, Dallas, Tex., USA

Prevention of infection after elective hysterectomy is a major concern for the gynecologic surgeon. Guidelines for prophylaxis were elegantly outlined by *Ledger* et al. [1] and were as follows:

(1) The operation should carry a significant risk of postoperative-site infection ... requiring systemic antibiotics or operative drainage.

(2) The operation should cause significant bacterial contamination.

(3) The antibiotic used for prophylaxis should have laboratory evidence of effectiveness against some of the contaminating microorganisms and demonstrable clinical effectiveness.

(4) The antibiotic should be present in the wound in effective concentrations at the time of incision.

(5) A short-term, low-toxicity regimen of antibiotics should be used.

(6) Antibiotics needed to combat resistant infections should be reserved and not used for prophylaxis.

(7) The benefits of prophylactic antibiotics must outweight the dangers of antibiotic use.

It is difficult to define 'significant' infection rate, since any infection is significant to both the patient who develops a major postoperative infection and to her surgeon. The infection rate observed and reported in a 1964 National Research Council study [2] was 5% for 'clean' cases and 10.8% for 'clean contaminated' cases. Hysterectomy was placed in the former category, but more realistically should have been placed in the latter category because of the normal flora of the vagina and endocervix that contaminate the operative site during surgery.

Flora

Most pelvic and abdominal incision infections after hysterectomy do develop in the hospital and are, for that reason, nosocomial according to strict definition. Perhaps they should realistically be considered community acquired, however, since pathogens recovered from infection sites are usually not hospital acquired, but rather are those brought into the hospital by the host, i.e. the lower reproductive tract flora. Although isolates may vary from one report to another, authors agree that the flora is polymicrobial containing both gram-positive and gram-negative aerobic and anaerobic bacteria [1, 3–22]. Preparation of the vagina prior to surgery reduces vaginal membrane bacterial count more efficiently than it does that in the endocervix [12, 17]. In one study, saline was as effective at accomplishing this goal as was povidone-iodine [18].

Several authors report that no significant differences in flora were detected in women who were pregnant, premenopausal on no hormones, premenopausal on oral contraceptives, or postmenopausal [9, 10, 19, 20]. *Thadepalli* et al. [22], however, reported increased recovery of *Escherichia coli* and *Bacteroides fragilis* during the proliferative phase of the menstrual cycle. Correspondingly, a higher incidence of postoperative infections was observed than when the surgery was performed during the secretory phase (31.6 vs. 18%). At least two reports [4, 13] have stressed the fact that recovery of bacteria prior to surgery or at uterine removal does not provide useful information regarding the prediction of subsequent postoperative infection. That has been our experience for both vaginal [23–26] and abdominal hysterectomy [25, 26]. Recovery of potential pathogens from the operative site after uterine removal is common [1, 4, 23, 25]. Postoperative alterations of bacterial flora observed were similar whether women were given antimicrobial prophylaxis or placebo when cultures were done prior to and following hysterectomy [6, 8, 15], making it difficult to ascribe such changes to prophylaxis.

Infection

Serious infections that develop following hysterectomy are polymicrobial [27–31], and anaerobes are significant both in early and late phases of these infections. Most isolates recovered from infection sites are those normally present in the lower reproductive tract. Identification of the true pathogens from such cultures is essentially impossible in most instances unless an abscess can be drained. This, combined with inaccessibility of infection site, make culturing the vaginal apex at infection a questionable endeavor. Septicemia is an uncommon occurrence in such infections, but, if positive, blood cultures will offer the surgeon significant information.

There is almost uniform agreement as to the definition of abdominal incision wound infection. Unfortunately, there are no uniform criteria for the diagnosis of postoperative pelvic infection. A term frequently appearing in gynecologic literature and equated with infection in many instances is 'febrile morbidity'. There are a minimum of nine different definitions for this diagnosis given by various authors. Temperature requirements, grace period after surgery, interval between temperature readings, and duration after surgery are variables in each definition. A statement frequently accompanying these temperature readings for febrile morbidity is, '...and obvious signs of clinical infection'. It is the experience of many, if not all, gynecologic surgeons that if one performs a speculum examination of the vagina between 48 and 96 h following a hysterectomy, it is common to see a purulent exudate in the vagina originating from the vaginal apex (cuff or surgical margin). The cuff is usually somewhat hyperemic and at bimanual examination, this area is indurated and frequently tender. These findings are present irrespective of the presence of temperature elevation or symptoms, but all would agree that these are, '...obvious signs of infection...'. It is the author's assumption, then, that all women develop 'infection' at the surgical vaginal margin, i.e. 'cuff cellulitis' after hysterectomy. Very few of these women, however, develop symptoms or signs of infection that require antimicrobial therapy. As high as 40% of women undergoing hysterectomy in the author's hospital have temperature measurements following surgery that meet criteria for febrile morbidity, yet do not require antimicrobial therapy.

Swartz [32] and *Shapiro* et al. [33] reported that febrile morbidity increased costs of health care. That has not been true in our patient population, which is almost entirely indigent. We have found it safe not to treat temperature elevation only. Women who develop a postoperative pelvic infection and require antimicrobial therapy in our hospital develop symptoms of pelvic and/or lower abdominal-back pain, and have tenderness at lower abdominal and pelvic examination that is usually asymmetric and maximal in the parametrial/adnexal areas. This we defined as pelvic cellulitis.

Falk and Bunkin [34] reported that 21.2% of 500 women developed febrile morbidity, yet only 8 (1.6%) infections were observed. *Ledger and Child* [35] reported that 54% of 3,564 women undergoing vaginal hysterectomy and 45% of 8,462 women undergoing abdominal hysterectomy were treated with antibiotics for postoperative infection. Postoperative fever $\geq$ 101 °F (38.4 °C) was reported in only 38 and 31%, respectively, however. *Gray* [36] reported an incidence of overall febrile morbidity of 20.8% for 2,421 women undergoing abdominal hysterectomy; wound infection rate, however, was only 0.4%. Infection rates or requirement for antibiotics reported by *Ledger* and *Gray* were significantly above those observed by The National Research Council [2], and underline the importance for the surgeon to know statistics for his/her patients in their respective hospitals. The percentages outlined by The National Research Council report, i.e. 5 and 10.8%, might be considered to be brackets for or at least the upper limit of the incidence of major infection following hysterectomy, whether it be pelvic or abdominal incision infection or a combination of the two. An infection rate higher than these should warrant at least a clinical trial of prophylaxis.

It is these major infections that prolong hospital stay and infrequently may require a second operative procedure if an abscess develops. The majority of pelvic infections, with and/or without an abscess, occur during the immediate postoperative period, but may occur after a completely benign postoperative course and discharge from the hospital. Pelvic cellulitis is much more common than abdominal incision infection following hysterectomy. Abscess development is uncommon but may occur, and drainage facilitates cure. If the abscess is immediately above the vaginal surgical margin, this can be accomplished easily. If not, a second operative procedure may be required although antimicrobial therapy alone usually results in cure. The advent of prophylaxis has been associated with a marked reduction in incidence of this significant complication. Although occurring much less frequently, infection in the abdominal incision prolongs hospital stay to a greater length and more significantly increases patient morbidity.

Prophylaxis Disadvantages

It is accepted that the prophylactic use of antibiotics presents several potential disadvantages. For that reason, it is important for the surgeon to know the infection rate in his patient population after vaginal and abdominal hysterectomy. Recognized potential adverse reactions associated with prolonged administration of antibiotics for prophylaxis include nonallergic toxicity, allergic reactions, alterations in host flora, alteration of antimicrobial resistance patterns in a hospital, induction of antibiotic-resistant infections before discharge from the hospital, prolonging onset of clinical signs of infection, and increased cost of hospitalization.

The longer an antibiotic is given, the more likely it is that problems will occur. Although these are infrequently serious, they may result in the patient's death [37]. Unexplained death has been reported after a single bolus injection of antimicrobial during anesthesia, as well [38]. Guidelines proposed by *Ledger* et al. [1] minimize these potential disadvantages.

Agent Selection

Selection of the agent to effectively and efficiently prevent infection should be made on the basis of the most frequent infecting organisms [1]. It has been established that infections are polymicrobial and anaerobes play a significant role. Guideline number 6 of *Ledger* et al. [1] recommends nonutilization of agents commonly selected to treat resistant infections, and treatment failures of initial medical therapy usually respond to the addition of anaerobic specific agents. Theoretically, the patient should be better protected by a prophylactic regimen possessing broader anaerobic coverage, as is seen with the newer cephalosporins and penicillins. Clinical trials shed light on this apparent dichotomy and will be reviewed later.

Administration

Many earlier studies evaluated multiple doses of antimicrobial administered over multiple days. Since there was a low incidence of toxic reactions, and since cost-containment was not given the complete attention as is currently encouraged, this practice was acceptable. Many investigators demonstrated a reduction in temperature elevations, significant infections, and hospital stay. With more awareness of adverse events and costs of medical care, periods of administration gradually shortened, and indeed, single-dose administration was proven to be as effective as multiple doses. Ideally, the agent selected should be in tissues that will be inoculated at the time of or shortly after contamination. *Burke* [39] showed that in an experimental animal model this was up to at least three hours following incision. Currently, adminstration is usually parenteral and given prior to the incision. Studies comparing route of administration with the same agent have not been reported. Obvious choices are intramuscularly on call to the operating room, usually one hour prior to incision, or intravenously on the operating room table. The former yields blood and tissue concentrations for prolonged periods while the latter results in higher concentrations in serum and pelvic tissues, but with fairly rapid elimination. We prefer the former. Mean cefoxitin concentrations ≥ 8.7 μg/g of myometrium, fallopian tube, or ovary have been observed through 199 min following a 2-gram intramuscular dose in our hospital [25]. *French* et al. [40] reported cefoxitin concentrations peaked at 30 μg/g tissue about 20 min after a 15-mg/kg intravenous dose, but were < 3 μg/g in pelvic tissue 2 h following the dose. Surgeon choice should prevail unless a particular route of administration is proven superior.

Vaginal Hysterectomy

In prospective controlled studies, the reported incidence of pelvic infection after vaginal hysterectomy without antibiotic prophylaxis varies from 12% [41] to 64% [42]. Several studies comparing an antibiotic to placebo or no drug showed that prophylaxis was not beneficial [41, 43–45]. These reports have been overwhelmed by the mass of prospective controlled studies showing efficacy of prophylaxis in preventing pelvic infection after vaginal hysterectomy, however [38, 42, 46–64]. The fact that several authors have reported that prophylaxis was not beneficial should not be overlooked, however. There are many practitioners who were performing vaginal hysterectomy when the 'prophylactic revolution' began. Their infection rates were low, hence the lack of necessity for prophylaxis for their patient populations. These data for such practitioners are - or should be - more meaningful than the 'local standard of care'.

It is difficult to identify 'universal' risk factors. *Shapiro* et al. [65] reported that younger age (not menopausal status), increased duration of operation, a clinic patient (rather than a private patient), and lack of prophylaxis were risk factors. *Taylor and Hansen* [66] and *Pratt and Galloway* (67] both reported increased morbidity, including infection, in younger women. *Hamod* et al. [68] reviewed the risk factors of age, menopausal status, phase of the menstrual cycle, and surgery-related factors, such as addition of anterior/posterior colporrhaphy. Some variables were related to infection for certain authors, but not for others. Age was not shown to be a factor in our hospital until our last study [69], in which older premenopausal women were at greater risk for infection. Our experience and that reviewed by *Hamod* et al. [68] has been that blood loss, surgical experience of the operator, and urethral catheterization were not related to infection. Increased operative time may or may not be a risk factor. This lack of uniformity of contribution to infection by these variables reported in the literature emphasizes again the importance of intimate knowledge by the surgeon of the risk factors - if any - for women having hysterectomy in his/her hospital under his/her care. Surgical technique is of obvious importance, but perhaps not as important as patients' host defence mechanisms, which are as yet not defined.

Regimens that have been evaluated and reported include penicillin [61], tetracycline [48], ampicillin [48, 52, 55], penicillin and streptomycin [46, 51, 55], carbenicillin [41], cephalothin [43, 47, 70], cefazolin [57–61, 63], cephradine [42, 64], cephaloridine [1, 49, 50, 58], cephaloridine plus cephalexin [1, 53, 54], cefoxitin [62], trimethoprim-sulfamethoxazole [44], metronidazole [45, 70], and chloramphenicol [46]. Very few comparative studies were being done initially, as most were placebo controlled. When comparative studies were reported, significant interregimen differences in efficacy were usually not found [48, 55, 58, 61, 70, 71]. Earlier studies involved the application of antibiotics for multiple days, but many single-dose regimens have proved effective [42, 44, 58, 70–73]. *Ledger* [74] recommended that *prophylaxis* should end in the recovery room. Not only are such regimens safer, they are also obviously more efficient in pharmacy and nursing unit space, nursing efforts and time, materials, and costs. A single, preoperative in-

Table I. Prophylaxis and vaginal hysterectomy in Parkland Memorial Hospital

Regimen-gram/dose	Reference	Dose(s)/h	Febrile morbidity %	Pelvic infection %	Mean hospital stay days
Retrospective (1971–1972)	75				
No drug (n = 244)		–	4.1	51.2	–
Cephalothin-1 (n = 30)		3/16	6.7	20	–
Retrospective (1974–1976)	76				
No drug (n = 41)		–	17.3	51	9.1
Cefazolin-1 (n = 194)		3/16	10.2	23	7.8
Prospective (1978–1979)	76				
Placebo (n = 49)		3/12	14.3	57	7.6
Cefoxitin-2 (n = 50)		3/12	14.0	8	4.8
Prospective[1] (1980)	77				
Doxycycline-0.2 (n = 26)		1/P	11.5	19.2	5.0
Cefamandole-2/1 (n = 25)		4/18	8.0	16.0	4.8
Prospective (1980)	un-				
Cefoxitin-2 (n = 111)	published	3/12	18.7	5.4	4.8
Prospective (1980)	un-				
Cefoxitin-2 (n = 44)	published	2/6	9.4	2.3	4.8
Cefoxitin-2 (n = 46)		3/12	18.8	6.5	5.2
Prospective (1980–1981)	23				
Moxalactam-1 (n = 93)		3/12	26.9	6.5	4.6
Cefazolin (n = 100)		3/12	17.0	5.0	4.5
Prospective[1] (1982)	24				
Cefoxitin-2 (n = 58)		1/P	17.2	1.7	4.4
Cefoxitin-2 (n = 54)		3/12	20.4	3.7	4.7
Prospective[1] (1982–1983)	69				
Ceftriaxone-1 (n = 57)		1/P	5.3	1.7	4.1
Cefazolin-1 (n = 60)		3/16	6.7	1.7	3.4

P = Preoperative only.
[1] Placebo blinded.

tramuscular dose of several antimicrobials has proved effective in our patient population, and is our preference.

Data from two retrospective and seven prospective studies conducted in our hospital since 1971 are summarized in table I with references.

Abdominal Hysterectomy

There is more controversy about requirement for and efficacy of prophylaxis for women undergoing elective abdominal hysterectomy. The same problems exist regarding definition of pelvic infection and the importance and meaning of temperature elevations. In addition, there is a second incision. This resulted in a definite increase in risk for infection according to *Shapiro* et al. [65]. The incidence of combined pelvic and wound infection rate in women given placebo or no drug reported in prospective comparative studies varies from 8% [78] to 50% [79, 80]. There are more studies indicating that prophylaxis does not significantly decrease the incidence of pelvic and wound infection [41, 56, 57, 61, 64, 79, 81–85] than were reported for vaginal hysterectomy. Many authors, however, reported that prophylaxis significantly reduced the incidence of major infection and/or shortened hospital stay compared to placebo or no drug [47, 57, 59, 60, 63, 79, 80, 86–91]. Antibiotics utilized were similar to those administered at vaginal hysterectomy, and dosing intervals and durations were similar, being longer in earlier studies. *Scarpignato* et al. [92] showed that 1 day of cefuroxime was as effective as 5 days of ampicillin and oxacillin, and *Kahn* et al. [93] reported that 2 doses of metronidazole were superior to placebo, but also that a single dose was not.

Data from a single retrospective study and five prospective studies conducted in women undergoing abdominal hysterectomy in our hospital since 1976 are summarized in table II, with references.

Abdominal versus Vaginal Hysterectomy

With the variability in requirements for antimicrobial prophylaxis at hysterectomy, we looked for uniformity in requirements for prophylaxis in a given hospital when studies comparing antibiotic to placebo

Table II. Prophylaxis and abdominal hysterectomy in Parkland Memorial Hospital

Regimen-gram/dose	Reference	Dose(s)/h	Febrile morbidity %	Pelvic/ abdominal infection %	Mean hospital stay days
Retrospective (1976–1978)	91				
No drug (n = 558)		–	9	64	6.8
Prospective (1979–1980)	91				
Placebo (n = 50)		3/12	34	32	6.4
Cefoxitin-2 (n = 50)		3/12	42	12	5.6
Prospective (1981)	91				
No drug (n = 74)		–	44	28	6.3
Cefoxitin-2 (n = 53)[1]		3/12	39	12	5.8
Prospective (1982)	25				
Cefoperazone-2 (n = 50)		3/12	28	6	5.7
Cefoxitin-2 (n = 51)		3/12	39	4	5.8
Prospective[2] (1982–1983)	69				
Ceftriaxone-1 (n = 54)		1/P	17	7	5.3
Cefazolin-1 (n = 54)		3/12	15	7	5.4
Prospective[2] (1983–1984)	un-published				
Cefoxitin-2 (n = 50)		1/P	40	4	5.5
Cefoxitin-2 (n = 50)		2/6	24	12	6.5
Cefoxitin-2 (n = 50)		3/12	24	4	5.4

P = Preoperative.
[1] High-risk group.
[2] Placebo blinded.

were reviewed. There were at least 3 authors who reported that prophylaxis did not significantly reduce the incidence of major infection for women undergoing vaginal or abdominal hysterectomy [41, 44, 45, 82]. Women given active agent in one study [41] had a hospital stay that was 3 days shorter than when placebo was given, however. At current costs for a day in the hospital, 3 days are significant! Several studies were found where antimicrobial prophylaxis significantly decreased the major infection rate for women undergoing vaginal hysterectomy, but not abdominal hysterectomy [53, 56, 57, 61, 64, 81, 85]. To complete the comparative, there were reports found, including those in our hospital, where prophylaxis significantly decreased the incidence of major infection irrespective of surgical approach [47, 59, 63, 76, 91]. No reports were found in which prophylaxis was beneficial for abdominal, but not vaginal hysterectomy.

New Agents

Newer cephalosporins and penicillins have increased activity against an expanded spectrum of potential pathogens including anaerobes. They have proved comparable in efficacy to combination regimens in the treatment of women with polymicrobial pelvic infections. Based on predicted pathogens recovered from infection sites, the normal assumption would be that the newer agents should offer better protection for prophylaxis than older agents. This premise has not been borne out by clinical trials involving either vaginal or abdominal hysterectomy [23, 25, 69, 94, 95]. It is possible that the newer agents might be more effective than older agents in certain groups of women such as those who have diabetes, carcinoma, or who are immunosuppressed, but such has not been proven.

We are currently evaluating single intramuscular doses of cefazolin (1 and 2 g), cefoxitin (2 g), and cefotaxime (1 g) in women undergoing vaginal hysterectomy to evaluate an efficacy 'generation-gap'. There is certainly a gap in the cost to our hospital per gram of agent, i.e.. $3.25 vs. $6.82 vs. $9.18, respectively. Patient costs per gram, are $13.61, $18.07, and $24.27, respectively. If practitioners are currently employing multiple doses of cefazolin over 24 h and obtain equal efficacy from a single dose of newer agent, the latter would be preferable in my opinion. Equal efficacy with single doses of each, however, should encourage the surgeon to use the former for prophylaxis and reserve the newer agent for therapy, where it is as effective and more efficient than combination therapy.

Antimicrobial prophylaxis for women undergoing elective abdominal and vaginal hysterectomy in our hospital saves an estimated $392,000 in health care costs annually. A single dose of several different regimens does this as effectively as multiple doses over 12–16 h. We must emphasize that these data are meaningful for our patient population only, which is theoretically at greatest risk, however, being primarily indigent. Each gynecologic surgeon must make these determinations in his/her own local setting.

References

1 Ledger, W.; Gee, C.; Lewis, W.: Guidelines for antibiotic prophylaxis in gynecology. Am. J. Obstet. Gynec. *121:* 1038–1045 (1975).

2 Ad Hoc Committee of the Committee on Trauma, Division of Medical Sciences, National Academy of Sciences, National Research Concil: Postoperatie wound infections. The influence of ultraviolet irradiation of the operating room and of various other factors. Ann. Surg. *160:* suppl., pp. 1–81 (1964).

3 Gorbach, S.; Menda, K.; Thadepalli, H.; Keith, L.: Anaerobic microflora of the cervix in healthy women. Am. J. Obstet. Gynec. *117:* 1053–1055 (1973).

4 George, J.; Ansbacher, R.; Otterson, W.; Rabey, F.: Prospective bacteriologic study of women undergoing hysterectomy. Obstet. Gynec., N.Y. *45:* 60–63 (1975).

5 Ohm, M.; Galask, R.: Bacterial flora of the cervix from 100 prehysterectomy patients. Am. J. Obstet. Gynec. *122:* 683–687 (1975).

6 Ohm, M.; Galask, R.: The effect of antibiotic prophylaxis on patients undergoing vaginal operations. II. Alterations of microbial flora. Am. J. Obstet. Gynec. *123:* 597–604 (1975).

7 Williams, D.; Knight, A.; King, H.; Harris, D.: The microbial flora of the vagina and its relationship to bacteriuria in diabetic and non-diabetic women. Br. J. Urol. *47:* 453–457 (1975).

8 Ohm, M.; Galask, R.: The effect of antibiotic prophylaxis on patients undergoing total abdominal hysterectomy. II. Alterations of microbial flora. Am. J. Obstet. Gynec. *125:* 448–454 (1976).

9 Tashjean, J.; Coulam, C.; Washington, J., II: Vaginal flora in asymptomatic women. Mayo Clin. Proc. *51:* 557–561 (1976).

10 Levison, M.; Corman, L.; Carrington, E.; Kaye, D.: Quantitative microflora of the vagina. Am. J. Obstet. Gynec. *127:* 80–85 (1977).

11 Onderdonk, A.; Polk, B.; Moon, N.; Goren, B.; Bartlett, J.: Methods for quantitative vaginal flora studies. Am. J. Obstet. Gynec. *128:* 777–781 (1977).

12 Osborne, N.; Wright, R.: Effect of preoperative scrub on the bacterial flora of the endocervix and vagina. Obstet. Gynec., N.Y. *50:* 148–151 (1977).

13 Grossman, J.; Adams, R.; Hierholzer, W. Jr.; Andriole, V.: Endometrial and vaginal cuff bacteria recovered at elective hysterectomy during a trial of antibiotic prophylaxis. Am. J. Obstet. Gynec. *130:* 312–316 (1978).

14 Bartlett, J.; Moon, N.; Goldstein, P.; Goren, B.; Onderdonk, A.; Polk, B.: Cervical and vaginal bacterial flora: Ecologic niches in the female lower genital tract. Am. J. Obstet. Gynec. *130:* 658–661 (1978).

15 Grossman, J., III; Adams, R.: Vaginal flora in women undergoing hysterectomy with antibiotic prophylaxis. Obstet. Gynec., N.Y. *53:* 23–26 (1979).

16 Hill, G.: How bacterial flora of the genital tract relates to infection. Contemp. Obstet/Gynec. *15:* 113-120 (1980).
17 Monif, G.; Thompson, J.; Stephens, H.; Baer, H.: Quantitative and qualitative effects of povidone-iodine liquid and gel on the aerobic and anaerobic flora of the female genital tract. Am. J. Obstet. Gynec. *137:* 432-438 (1980).
18 Amstey, M.; Jones, A.: Preparation of the vagina for surgery. J. Am. med. Ass. *245:* 839-841 (1981).
19 Larsen, B.; Goplerud, C.; Petzold, C.; Ohm-Smith, M.; Galask, R.: Effect of estrogen treatment on the genital tract flora of postmenopausal women. Obstet. Gynec., N.Y. *60:* 20-24 (1982).
20 Mehta, P.: Vaginal flora, a dynamic ecosystem. J. reprod. Med. *27:* 455-458 (1982).
21 Spence, M.; Blanco, L.; Patel, J.; Brokman, M.: A comparative evaluation of vaginal, cervical, and peritoneal flora in normal, healthy women. A preliminary report. Sexually transm. Dis. *9:* 37-40 (1982).
22 Thadepalli, H.; Savage, E., Jr.; Salem, F.; Roy, I.; Davidson, E. Jr.: Cyclic changes in cervical microflora and their effect on infections following hysterectomy. Gynecol. obstet. Invest. *14:* 176-183 (1982).
23 Hemsell, D.; Hemsell, P.; Nobles, B.; Heard, M.; Bawdon, R.: Moxalactam versus cefazolin prophylaxis for vaginal hysterectomy. Am. J. Obstet. Gynec. *147:* 379-385 (1983).
24 Hemsell, D.; Heard, M.; Nobles, B.; Hemsell, P.: Single-dose cefoxitin prophylaxis for premenopausal women undergoing vaginal hysterectomy. Obstet. Gynec., N.Y. *63:* 285-290 (1984).
25 Hemsell, D.; Johnson, E.; Bawdon, R.; Hemsell, P.; Heard, M.; Nobles, B.: Cefoperazone and cefoxitin prophylaxis for abdominal hysterectomy. Obstet. Gynec., N.Y. *63:* 467-472 (1984).
26 Heard, M.; Bawdon,R.; Hemsell, D.; Nobles, B.: Susceptibility profiles of potential aerobic and anaerobic pathogens isolated from hysterectomy patients. Am. J. Obstet. Gynec. *149:* 133-143 (1984).
27 Swenson, R.; Michaelson, T.; Daly, M.; Spaulding, E.: Anaerobic bacterial infections of the female genital tract. Obstet. Gynec., N.Y. *42:* 538-541 (1973).
28 Thadepalli, H.; Gorbach, S.; Keith, L.: Anaerobic infections of the female genital tract. Bacteriologic and therapeutic aspects. Am. J. Obstet. Gynec. *117:* 1034-1040 (1973).
29 Sweet, R.: Anaerobic infections of the female genital tract. Am. J. Obstet. Gynec. *122:* 891-901 (1975).
30 Bartlett, J.: Anaerobic infections of the pelvis. Clin. Obstet. Gynec. *21:* 351-360 (1979).
31 Sweet, R., Yonekura, M.; Hill, G.; Gibbs, R.; Eschenbach, D.: Appropriate use of antibiotics in serious obstetric and gynecologic infections. Am. J. Obstet. Gynec. *146:* 719-739 (1983).
32 Swartz, W.: Prophylaxis of minor febrile and major infectious morbidity following hysterectomy. Obstet. Gynec., N.Y. *54:* 284-285 (1979).
33 Shapiro, M.; Schoenbaum, S.; Tager, I.; Muñoz, A.; Polk, B.: Benefit-cost analysis of antimicrobial prophylaxis in abdominal and vaginal hysterectomy. J. Am. med., Ass. *249:* 1290-1294 (1983).

34 Falk, H.; Bunkin, I.: A study of 500 vaginal hysterectomies. Am. J. Obstet. Gynec. *52:* 623-630 (1946).

35 Ledger, W.; Child, M.: The hospital care of patients undergoing hysterectomy: An analysis of 12,026 patients from the Professional Activity Study. Am. J. Obstet. Gynec. *117:* 423-433 (1973).

36 Gray, L.: Open cuff method of abdominal hysterectomy. Obstet. Gynec., N.Y. *46:* 42-46 (1975).

37 Ledger, W.: Puttler, O.: Death from pseudomembranous enterocolitis. Obstet. Gynec., N.Y. *45:* 609-613 (1975).

38 Clement, J.: Prophylactic antibiotics in hysterectomy. N. Carol. med. J. *36:* 542-543 (1975).

39 Burke, J.: The effective period of preventive antibiotic action in experimental incisions and dermal lesions. Surgery *50:* 161-168 (1961).

40 French, M.; Quintiliani, R.; Nightingale, C.; Russo, J.: Serum and tissue concentrations of cefoxitin and cefamandole in women undergoing hysterectomy. Obstet. Gynec., N.Y. *61:* 42-47 (1983).

41 Roberts, J.; Homesley, H.: Low-dose carbenicillin prophylaxis for vaginal and abdominal hysterectomy. Obstet. Gynec., N.Y. *52:* 83-87 (1978).

42 Mendelson, J.; Portnoy, J.; De Saint Victor, J.; Gelfand, M.: Effect of single and multidose cephradine prophylaxis on infectious morbidity of vaginal hysterectomy. Obstet. Gynec., N.Y. *53:* 31-35 (1979).

43 Bivens, M.; Neufeld, J.; McCarty, W.: The prophylactic use of Keflex and Keflin in vaginal hysterectomy. Am. J. Obstet. Gynec. *122:* 169-175 (1975).

44 Mathews, D.; Agarwal, V.; Gordon, A.; Cooper, J.: A double-blind trial of single-dose chemoprophylaxis with co-trimoxazole during vaginal hysterectomy and repair. Br. J. Obstet. Gynaec. *86:* 737-740 (1979).

45 Vincelette, J.; Finkelstein, F.; Aoki, F.; Ti, T.; Ogilvie, R.; Richard, G.; Seymour, R.: Double blind trial of perioperative intravenous metronidazole prophylaxis for abdominal and vaginal hysterectomy. Surgery *93:* 185-189 (1983).

46 Goosenberg, J., Emich, J., Schwarz, R.: Prophylactic antibiotics in vaginal hysterectomy. Am. J. Obstet. Gynec. *105:* 503-506 (1969).

47 Allen, J.; Rampone, J.; Wheeless, C.: Use of a prophylactic antibiotic in elective major gynecologic operations. Obstet. Gynec., N.Y. *39:* 218-224 (1972).

48 Bolling, D., Jr.; Plunkett, G.: Prophylactic antibiotics for vaginal hysterectomies. Obstet. Gynec., N.Y. *41:* 689-692 (1973).

49 Ledger, W.; Sweet, R.; Headington, J.: Prophylactic cephaloridine in the prevention of postoperative pelvic infections in premenopausal women undergoing vaginal hysterectomy. Am. J. Obstet. Gynec. *115:* 766-774 (1973).

50 Breedon, J.; Mayo, J.: Low dose prophylactic antibiotics in vaginal hysterectomy. Obstet. Gynec., N.Y. *43:* 379-385 (1974).

51 Harralson, J.; Nagell, J., Jr. van; Roddick, J.; Sprague, A.: The effect of prophylactic antibiotics on pelvic infections following vaginal hysterectomy. Am. J. Obstet. Gynec. *120:* 1046-1049 (1974).

52 Jackson, C.; Amstey, M.: Prophylactic ampicillin therapy for vaginal hysterectomy. Surg. Gynec. Obstet. *141:* 755-757 (1975).

53 Ohm, M.; Galask, R.: The effect of antibiotic prophylaxis on patients undergoing vaginal operations. I. The effect on morbidity. Am. J. Obstet. Gynec. *123:*590-596 (1975).

54 Forney, J.; Morrow, C.; Townsend, D.; DiSaia, P.: Impact of cephalosporin prophylaxis on conization - vaginal hysterectomy morbidity. Am. J. Obstet. Gynec. *125:* 100-103 (1976).

55 Glover, M.; Nagell, J., Jr. van: The effect of prophylactic ampicillin on pelvic infection following vaginal hysterectomy. Am. J. Obstet. Gynec. *126:* 385-388 (1976).

56 Mayer, W.; Gordon, M.; Rothbard, M.: Prophylactic antibiotics. Use in hysterectomy. N.Y. St. J. Med. *76:* 2144-2147 (1976).

57 Swartz, W.; Tanaree, P.: T-tube suction drainage and/or prophylactic antibiotics. A randomized study of 451 hysterectomies. Obstet. Gynec., N.Y. *47:* 665-670 (1976).

58 Lett, W.; Ansbacher, R.; Davison, B.; Otterson, W.: Prophylactic antibiotics for women undergoing vaginal hysterectomy. J. reprod. Med. *19:* 51-54 (1977).

59 Holman, J.; McGowan, J.; Thompson, J.: Perioperative antibiotics in major elective gynecologic surgery. South. med. J. 71: 417-420 (1978).

60 Jennings, R.: Prophylactic antibiotics in vaginal and abdominal hysterectomy. South. med. J. *71:* 251-254 (1978).

61 Grossman, J.; III; Greco, T.; Minkin, M.; Adams, R.; Hierholzer, W., Jr.; Andriole, V.: Prophylactic antibiotics in gynecologic surgery. Obstet. Gynec., N.Y. *53:* 537-544 (1979).

62 Mickal, A.; Curole, D.; Lewis, C.: Cefoxitin Sodium: Double-blind vaginal hysterectomy prophylaxis in premenopausal patients. Obstet. Gynec., N.Y. *56:* 222-225 (1980).

63 Polk, B.; Tager, I.; Shapiro, M.; Goren-White, B.; Goldstein, P.; Schoenbaum, S.: Randomised clinical trial of perioperative cefazolin in preventing infection after hysterectomy. Lancet *i:* 437-440 (1980).

64 Stage, A.; Glover, D.; Vaughn, J.: Low-dose cephradine prophylaxis in obstetric and gynecologic surgery. J. reprod. Med. *27:* 113-119 (1982).

65 Shapiro, M.; Muñoz, A.; Tager, I.; Schoenbaum, S.; Polk, B.: Risk factors for infection at the operative site after abdominal or vaginal hysterectomy. New Engl. J. Med. *307:* 1661-1666 (1982).

66 Taylor, E.; Hansen, R.: Morbidity following vaginal hysterectomy. Obstet. Gynec., N.Y. *17:* 346-348 (1961).

67 Pratt, J.; Galloway, J.: Vaginal hysterectomy in patients less than 36 or more than 60 years of age. Am. J. Obstet. Gynec. *93:* 812-821 (1965).

68 Hamod, K.; Spence, M.; King, T.: Prophylactic antibiotics in vaginal hysterectomy. A review. Obstet. Gynec. Surv. *37:* 207-216 (1982).

69 Hemsell, D.; Hemsell, P.; Nobles, B.; Heard, M.; Bawdon, R.: Ceftriaxone and cefazolin prophylaxis for hysterectomy. Surg. Gynec. Obstet. (in press).

70 Hamod, K.; Spence, M.; Rosenshein, N.; Dillon, M.: Single-dose and multidose prophylaxis in vaginal hysterectomy: a comparison of sodium cephalothin and metronidazole. Am. J. Obstet. Gynec. *136:* 976-979 (1980).

71 Jacobson, J.; Hebertson, R.; Kasworm, E.: Comparison of ceforanide and cephalothin prophylaxis for vaginal hysterectomies. Antimicrob. Agents Chemother. *22:* 643-647 (1982).

72 Lander, J.; Steigrad, S.: Single dose preoperative prophylactic antibiotic in vaginal hysterectomy. Aust. N.Z.J. Obstet. Gynaec. *18:* 73-77 (1978).

73 Hemsell, D.; Menon, M.; Friedman, A.: Ceftriaxone and cefazolin for prevention of infection following vaginal hysterectomy. Am. J. Surg. (in press).

74 Ledger, W.: Prevention, diagnosis, and treatment of postoperative infections. Obstet. Gynecol. *55:* suppl., pp. 203S–206S (1980).
75 Scott, J.: Pelvic infections following vaginal hysterectomy. Hosp. Prac. *8:* 101–110 (1973).
76 Hemsell, D.; Cunningham, F.; Kappus, S.; Nobles, B.: Cefoxitin for prophylaxis in premenopausal women undergoing vaginal hysterectomy. Obstet. Gynec., N.Y. *56:* 629–634 (1980).
77 Hemsell, D.; Hemsell, P.; Nobles, B.: Doxycycline and cefamandole prophylaxis for premenopausal women undergoing vaginal prophylaxis. Surg. Gynec. Obstet. (submitted, 1984).
78 Creasman, W.; Hill, G.; Weed, J.; Gall, S.: A trial of prophylactic cefamandole in-extended gynecologic surgery. Obstet. Gynec., N.Y. *59:* 309–314 (1982).
79 Appelbaum, P.; Moodley, J.; Chatterton, S.; Cowan, D.; Africa, C.: Metronidazole in the prophylaxis and treatment of anaerobic infection. S. Afr. med. J. *54:* 703–706 (1978).
80 Appelbaum, P.; Moodley, J.; Chatterton, S.; Cowan, D.; Africa, C.: Tinidazole in the prophylaxis and treatment of anaerobic infection. Chemotherapy *26:* 145–151 (1980).
81 Ohm, M.; Galask, R.: The effect of antibiotic prophylaxis on patients undergoing total abdominal hysterectomy. I. Effect on morbidity. Am. J. Obstet. Gynec. *125:* 442–447 (1976).
82 Mathews, D.; Ross, H.; Cooper, J.: A double-blind trial of single-dose chemoprophylaxis with co-trimoxazole during total abdominal hysterectomy. Br. J. Obstet. Gynaec. *84:* 894–897 (1977).
83 Duff, P.: Antibiotic prophylaxis for abdominal hysterectomy. Obstet. Gynec., N.Y. *60:* 25–29 (1982).
84 Popkin, D.; Martinez, L.; Carswell, G.: Metronidazole in the prophylaxis of anaerobic infections in gynecologic surgery. Surgery *93:* 180–184 (1983).
85 Savage, E.; Thadepalli, H.; Rambhatla, K.; Roy, I.; Davidson, E., Jr.: Minocycline prophylaxis in elective hysterectomy. J. reprod. Med. *29:* 81–87 (1984).
86 Sengupta, B.; Wynter, H.; Hall, J.; Ramchander, R.; Alexis, A.; Zamah, N.; Gajraj, K.: Prophylactic antibiotic in elective gynaecological and obstetrical major surgery. Int. J. Gynaec. Obstet. *14:* 417–424 (1976).
87 Mathews, D.; Agarwal, V.; Ross, H.: A randomized controlled trial of a short course of cephaloridine in the prevention of infection after abdominal hysterectomy. Br. J. obstet. Gynaec. *85:* 381–385 (1978).
88 Wheeless, C.; jr.; Dorsey, J.; Wharton, L., Jr.: An evaluation of prophylactic doxycycline in hysterectomy patients. J. reprod. Med. *21:* 146–150 (1978).
89 Itskovitz, J.; Fisher, M.; Urbach, J.; Brandes, J.: The effect of a short-term course of antibiotic prophylaxis on patients undergoing total abdominal hysterectomy. Eur. J. Obstet. Gynaec. reprod. Biol. *11:* 101–107 (1980).
90 Karhunen, M.; Kosleka, O.; Hannelin, M.: Single dose of tinidazole in prophylaxis of infections following hysterectomy. Br. J. Obstet. Gynaec. *87:* 70–72 (1980).
91 Hemsell, D.; Reisch, J.; Nobles, B.; Hemsell, P.: Prevention of major infection following elective abdominal hysterectomy: Individual determination required. Am. J. Obstet. Gynec. *147:* 520–528 (1983).

92 Scarpignato, C.; Labruna, C.; Condemi, V.; Mansani, F.: Comparative efficacy of two different regimens of antibiotic prophylaxis in total abdominal hysterectomy. Pharmatherapeutica *2:* 450–455 (1980).
93 Kahn, M.; Begg, H.; Frampton, J.; Hughes, T.: A comparative study of the prophylactic effect of one dose and two doses of intravenous metronidazole therapy in gynaecological surgery. Scand. J. infect. Dis. *26:* suppl. pp. 115–117 (1980).
94 Wideman, G.; Matthijssen, C.: Comparative efficacy of cefotaxime and cefazolin as prophylaxis against infections following elective hysterectomy. Clin. Ther. *5:* suppl. A, pp. 67–73 (1982).
95 Roy, S.; Wilkins, J.: Comparison of cefotaxime with cefazolin for prophylaxis of vaginal or abdominal hysterectomy. Clin. Ther *5:* suppl. A pp. 74–82 (1982).

D.L. Hemsell, MD, Department of Obstetrics and Gynecology,
University of Texas Health Science Center at Dallas,
Southwestern Medical School,
Parkland Memorial Hospital, Dallas, TX 75235 (USA)

Antibiot. Chemother., vol. 33, pp. 90–113 (Karger, Basel 1985)

Prevention of Infection in Neutropenic Bone Marrow Transplant Patients

T.R. Rogers

Department of Medical Microbiology, Westminster Medical School, London, UK

Introduction

Bone marrow transplantation (BMT) is being increasingly undertaken as a curative procedure in patients suffering from otherwise fatal diseases such as leukaemia and aplastic anaemia. Most frequently, marrow is obtained from a healthy family donor and given to the patient as an allogeneic transplant, but occasionally the patient's own marrow is harvested and stored only to be returned at some later date as an autograft. Since the pioneering days of almost 30 years ago when BMT was first attempted in man [43, 65, 76], it has become clear that there are some critical requirements for a successful outcome. Most important among these is the need for immunological compatibility between donor and recipient tissues in order to prevent fatal acute graft-versus-host disease (GVHD). The advent of accurate tissue typing, with the use of the HLA system, opened up new opportunities for attempting BMT in a variety of clinical disorders, and throughout the 1970s valuable experience was gained in applying transplantation to the treatment of acute leukaemias [5, 58, 75], aplastic anaemias [22, 35, 38] and inborn errors of metabolism [33]. Presently, transplants are most often carried out between fully HLA matched siblings; however, as this desirable situation does not always exist, attempts have been made in recent years to use either unrelated HLA matched or related HLA mismatched donors.

This experience has revealed the major importance of infection as an additional cause of morbidity and death after BMT [13, 69, 92]. The

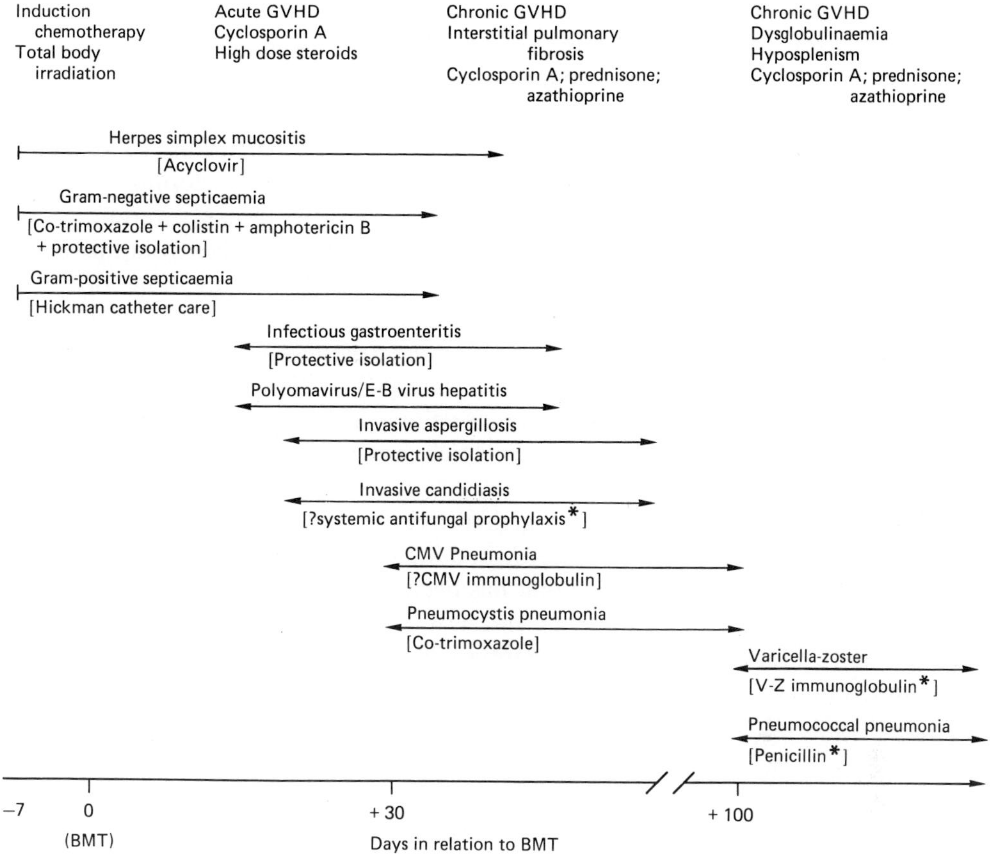

Fig. 1. Approximate risk periods for infectious complications during bone marrow transplantation and appropriate preventive measures. Top column shows factors which at various time periods increase the risk of infection. *Indicated for selected patients only.

nature and severity of infectious complications each depend on the type of transplant and immunosuppression used, the patient's age and underlying disease, and on the time at which they occur following a BM graft. As a result of this experience it is now apparent that certain time periods exist after BMT during which there is a particular risk of acquiring infections with specific agents (fig. 1) and of developing related clinical problems [48]. In the first few weeks after transplantation, infections arise primarily as a result of neutropenia and also from the effects of the preparative immunosuppression. From the time of engraftment to 3 or 4 months after transplant, the major problem is interstitial pneumonia which occurs most frequently in irradiated patients and carries a high mortality rate [51]. Patients who survive beyond this time may develop late infections [2, 18] owing to the continuing state of immune deficiency which may persist for up to a year or more.

A recent meeting brought together investigators from major transplant centres in Europe and the United States [88] and helped to illustrate the differing experience that has been gained in dealing with infection in this group of patients, and how various strategies have been developed for its control. This chapter will attempt to assess the merits and rationale of these infection-prevention measures and will make particular reference to the neutropenic period.

Risk Factors for Infection in the Early Post-Transplant Period

The association between neutropenia and an increased risk of infection has long been recognised [95], and most of the detailed studies on this subject have been carried out in patients undergoing chemotherapy for haematological malignancies. One of the earliest of these [9] assessed the relationship between the degree and duration of neutropenia and the incidence and severity of infection. An increased incidence of infection was found in those acute leukaemia patients whose neutrophil counts fell below $1.5 \times 10^9/l$, and a fatal outcome was most likely to occur in the face of profound and prolonged neutropenia. Infected patients who failed to mount a neutrophil response, and especially those whose disease was in relapse, fared worst of all. These important observations have been confirmed by other investigators [72].

The conditioning regimens used to prevent graft rejection are given in the few days before BMT and usually lead to a profound neutropenia by the fifth day after transplant. The recovery of bone marrow function coincident with successful engraftment is likely to take place by the beginning of the fourth week [48]. It is therefore during these first 3–4 weeks that the chance of developing major bacterial infection is greatest. Despite the return to normal neutropil numbers, qualitative abnormalities in white cell function have been reported to occur, particularly in the face of active GVHD [21], and may account for the sustained susceptibility to bacterial infection in the succeeding weeks post-transplant. Both aplastic anaemia patients who are neutropenic pre-transplant, and those who reject the transplanted marrow, will experience the most prolonged duration of neutropenia and are at greatest risk in this respect [71]. It is in this situation that invasive fungal infection is most likely to occur.

Various schedules have been devised for conditioning of the patient before transplant and these will, to varying degrees, depress the cell-mediated immunity of the host [46]. This in turn may trigger a reactivation of certain latent viruses which themselves are immunosuppressive [74]. The situation is likely to be aggravated by the appearance of acute GVHD and by the use of steroids or other chemotherapy for its control [37].

Total body irradiation is usually given to leukaemia patients shortly before transplant in order to eradicate residual tumour cells, and is associated with the development of interstitial pneumonia in the succeeding 3 months or so [48, 51]. It is less well appreciated that both this form of irradiation and other conditioning regimens can damage the intestinal and other mucosal surfaces [36] and this might create a portal of entry for bacteraemic organisms. A further effect which has become better recognised is the impaired absorption of certain drugs that have been incorporated into oral prophylactic regimens used during neutropenia [29].

A number of additional measures have become an established component of the support given to the neutropenic patient. These include the use of an indwelling right atrial catheter which provides continuous access to the circulation [32]. The widespread use of the Hickman catheter for this purpose illustrates how valuable it is for management but, at the same time, localised skin infection and septicaemia may complicate its use. White cell transfusions have been found to be

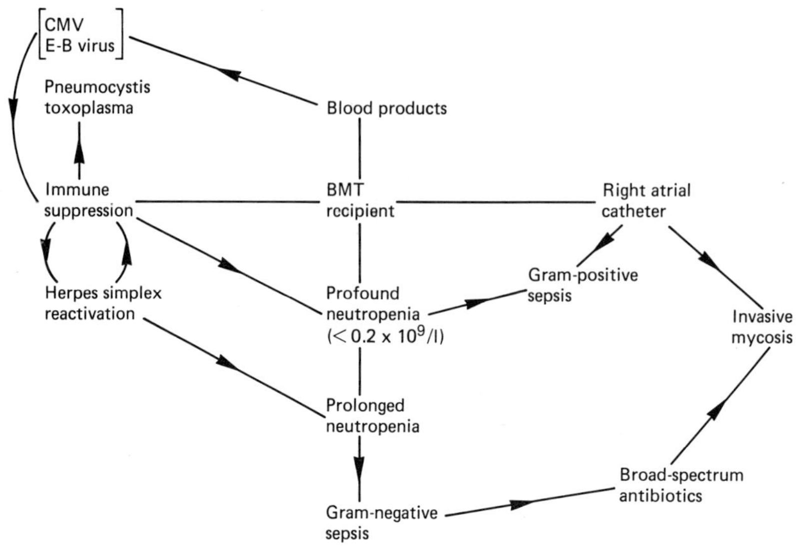

Fig. 2. Interplay of patient risk factors and related infectious complications after bone marrow transplantation.

of value both in the prevention [14] and treatment [73] of infection during neutropenia. However, the transmission of cytomegalovirus is a well-recognised hazard of this practice and has limited its application [12].

From experience of these events it is apparent that a subtle interplay can take place between these various risk factors, as have been outlined above, so that the occurrence of one may trigger superadded infection (fig. 2).

Infections

Septicaemia

Fever is a frequent occurrence in the early weeks after transplantation and in the absence of signs of acute GVHD or localised infection, the likelihood of septicaemia must be seriously considered. Laboratory confirmation, with the isolation of a causative organism, is likely to be achieved in less than half of the clinically documented episodes even with the best facilities available [57]. From the early studies in BMT patients, the pattern of infecting organisms was similar to that seen in patients undergoing conventional treatment for leukaemia with a predominance of septicaemias due to gram-negative organisms and an incidence of over 50%. Although infections with enterobacteria, and particularly *Pseudomonas aeruginosa*, still carry a high mortality rate, more recent reviews have drawn attention to the growing frequency of *Staphylococcus epidermidis* bacteraemias [8]. This change has been temporally related to the introduction of right atrial catheters, although the withdrawal of vancomycin from gut decontamination regimens has been offered as an alternative explanation [86]. Certain serotypes of corynebacteria [70] and members of the viridans streptococci [15, 31] have also been reported as 'new' pathogens in a similar context. An additional factor for streptococcal bacteraemia may be ulceration of the oropharyngeal mucosa which occurs with herpes simplex mucositis. Beyond the period of neutropenia, septicaemia occasionally occurs, but when neutropenia persists antibiotic-resistant bacteraemia and especially invasive candidiasis [45] are more likely to present.

Localised Skin Infection

This may precede the onset of septicaemia and often involves the wound exit site of the indwelling venous catheter. *S. epidermidis* is most often implicated in these infections. Persistent infection accompanied by septicaemia or metastatic lesions may necessitate premature removal of the catheter [63].

Embolic lesions in the skin are sometimes seen as a complication of staphylococcal septicaemia while gangrenous ulcers are a pathognomonic sign of advanced *Pseudomonas aeruginosa* infection.

Herpes simplex Mucositis

Reactivation of herpes simplex virus occurs in at least 80% of BMT patients with latent infection [48]. Apart from the troublesome mucosal ulceration that often occurs as a feature of this disease, attention has recently been drawn to the further complication of myelosuppression with its additional associated problems [59].

Reactivation of latent papovavirus infection has been reported to occur in over 50% of leukaemic BMT recipients in some of whom transient hepatic dysfunction may result [53].

Intestinal Infections

Diarrhoea may be drug induced, due to GVHD or the result of infection. Several viruses and also *Clostridium difficile* have been found to be associated with a high morbidity in this setting [78, 94] and nosocomial spread may be an important factor in determining the frequency of these infections [62]. Atypical presentations of clostridial colitis have recently been reported in neutropenic patients [39].

Intestinal candidiasis is most likely to arise in patients with underlying GVH involving the intestinal tract. Oesophagitis is another manifestation of candidal infection and usually occurs as a progression of oro-pharyngeal infection.

Pulmonary Infections

Interstitial pneumonia is one of the most serious complications arising after BMT. The incidence is highest where irradiation forms part of the conditioning regimen and it has been reported to occur in up to 40% of patients between 1 and 4 months after BMT [52]. In studies where lung biopsy has been carried out to confirm the diagnosis of pneumonia, CMV has been demonstrated in nearly half of proven cases [51]. Other respiratory viruses have been implicated but as a result of successful prophylaxis with co-trimoxazole *Pneumocystis carinii* has become a rare cause [34].

Aspergillus spp. may cause invasive disease, especially in patients suffering prolonged neutropenia [24] and has proved difficult both to diagnose early and treat effectively.

Preventive Measures

From the preceding section it is evident that the neutropenic BMT patient is at great risk of experiencing a serious infective episode following transplantation, and in a recent study at least one major infection was documented in 75% of leukaemic transplants [4]. Infecting organisms may originate either from the patients' own 'endogenous' flora, from such sites as the bowel, oropharynx, skin and in the female the lower genital tract, or from 'exogenous' sources notably staff and other patients, the inanimate environment, blood products (including the transplanted marrow) and food. Over the years, preventive measures have evolved which are based on the principles of antibiotic suppres-

Table I. Preventive measures in patients undergoing BMT

Out-patient visit
Dental examination
Chest, sinus X-rays
Baseline antibody studies for CMV, herpes simplex, varicella-zoster, pneumocystis
Urine culture for CMV (in < 5 year olds)
Admission 1 week pre-BMT
Insertion of right atrial catheter
Perform surveillance cultures
Begin oral antifungal prophylaxis
Begin oral chemoprophylaxis and protective isolation 1–3 days before induction regimen
Until engraftment (granulocytes > $0.5 \times 10^9/l$)
Oral prophylaxis and isolation continued
Surface decontamination; 'clean' food cooked preferably on unit, and sterile canned food
Weekly surveillance cultures
Active treatment for GVHD
Continue protective isolation (preferably with filtered air under positive pressure)
Day 100/discharge
Zoster immune globulin to seronegative patients and continue monthly up to one year post-BMT

sion of patients' resident organisms, combined with protective isolation and attention to diet to prevent exogenous infection. Accordingly, many units have adopted procedures similar to those outlined in table I for management of the BMT patient from the time of admission until discharge from hospital.

Measures Undertaken Pre-Transplant

Ideally, the patient should be admitted a week or more before BMT. Baseline sera will have been obtained at a previous out-patient visit for screening for hepatitis B, CMV, other herpes viruses and Pneumocystis. X-rays of teeth and sinuses help to outrule occult sepsis, and

Table II. Recent examples of chemoprophylactic regimens used in neutropenic patients

Reference	Oral regimen	Number of doses per 24 h	Topical skin + mucosal regimen	Other measures
Watson et al. [89]	neomycin 500 mg	2		
	colistin 1.5×10^6 U	2		
	or trimethoprim 160 mg	2		room with
	sulphamethoxazole 800 mg	2		positive pressure
	+ nystatinelixir 100,000 U	2		filtered air
	nystatin tabs. 500,000 U	2		+
	amphotericin B lozenges 10 mg	4		'pathogen-free' diet
	amphotericin B tabs 200 mg	4		
Guiot et al. [26]	neomycin 250 mg	4	3% gentamicin to oropharynx am-	LAF or single room
	polymixin 100 mg	4	photericin B/neomycin/polymixin	isolation
	nalidixic acid 1 g	4	in orabase to mouth or vulva and	
	amphotericin B 250 mg	4	vagina 0.02% chlorhexidine to skin	
De Vries Hospers et al. [20]	nalidixic acid 2 g	4		
	or trimethoprim 160 mg sulphamethoxazole 800 mg	3		
	or polymixin 200 mg	4		
	+ amphotericin B 2 g	1		

Table II (cont.)

Reference	Oral regimen	Number of doses per 24 h	Topical skin + mucosal regimen	Other measures
Wade et al. [85]	trimethoprim 160 mg	2	chlorhexidine skin scrub	
	sulphamethoxazole 800 mg	2		cooked food
	nystatin 1×10^6 U	6	povidone iodine swabbing of	
	or gentamicin 200 mg	1	axilla, groins, perineum	
	nystatin 4×10^6 U tablets	1		
	nystatin 1×10^6 U suspension	6		
Storring et al. [72]	framycetin 500 mg	4	1% chlorhexidine nasal cream	single room isolation
	colistin 1.5×10^6 U	4	0.02% chlorhexidine mouth wash,	+
	nystatin 1×10^6 U	4	ears, nose, throat	'pathogen-free' food
			1% obstetric cream	
Lindgren [42]	tobramycin 80 mg	3	chlorhexidine soap to skin	
	vancomycin 250 mg	3	vancomycin/neomycin/polymixin	
	polymixin 750 mg	3	cream to nasopharynx	
	nystatin 3×10^6 U	3	polymixin/bacitracin/neomycin	sterile food
			to axilla, groins, ears, nose, rectum	+
			povidone iodine	LAF
			vaginal douche	

Table III. Findings of chemoprophylactic studies in neutropenic BMT recipients

Reference	Study group (number of patients)	Study period	Study design	Result					
				septi-caemia	major local infection	infective death	herpes simplex infection	CMV infection	candidal infection
Navari et al. [50]	aplasia (101)	day 0 to engraftment	LAF + non-absorbable antibiotics	2	1	0			
			vs. granulocytes	4	5	0			
			vs. single room isolation	11	6	1			
Buckner et al. [11]	acute leukaemia (161)	day 0 to engraftment	LAF + non-absorbable antibiotics	18	11	4			
			vs. granulocytes	16	11	3			
Buckner et al. [10]	acute leukaemia; aplasia (90)	day 0 to + 50	LAF + non-absorbable antibiotics	10	3	0			
			vs. single room isolation	23	22	1			

Table III (cont.)

Reference	Study group (number of patients)	Study period	Study design	Result					
				septi-caemia	major local infection	infective death	herpes simplex infection	CMV infection	candidal infection
Clift et al. [14]	leukaemia; aplasia (69)	while peripheral granulocytes $< 0.2 \times 10^9/l$	granulocytes vs. control	0 10	2 7	0 4			
Prentice [59]	acute leukaemia (20)	day 0 to granulocytes $> 0.5 \times 10^9/l$	acyclovir vs. placebo				0 5	1 0	
Gluckman et al. [25]	leukaemia; aplasia (39)	day 0 to +35	acyclovir vs. placebo				0 13	0 7	
Kraemer et al. [40]	leukaemia (38)	day when peripheral granulocytes $> 0.5 \times 10^9/l$ to day + 100	adenine arabinoside vs. control					12 7	
Hann et al. [28]	leukaemia; aplasia (19)	while granulocytes $< 1 \times 10^9/l$	ketoconazole vs. amphotericin B + nystatin						5 9

carious teeth should be removed. If there is evidence of sinusitis, surgical drainage and microbiological examination are indicated. The sinuses have been identified as an important source of aspergillus [6] and amphotericin wash-outs can be considered if *Aspergillus* spp. is recovered in surveillance cultures.

In the week before BMT a right atrial catheter is inserted using full surgical aseptic technique, chemoprophylaxis is started, and the patient is introduced into a protective environment.

Chemoprophylaxis

The application of antibiotics for prophylaxis of bacterial infection during BMT has to be considered in the context of similar efforts in neutropenic patients undergoing conventional therapy for haematological and other malignancies, and also in the light of observations made in animal studies. The bowel is acknowledged as being the principal source of septicaemia organisms, both from the patient's own flora and from colonizing bacteria originating from exogenous sources. In early studies, so-called 'gut decontamination' regimens which consisted of combinations of oral non-absorbable antibiotics were employed to suppress the bowel flora and these proved particularly effective when combined with a protective environment [41, 66]. However, the work of *Van der Waaij* et al. [81] in animals drew attention to the fact that retention of the anaerobic flora of the bowel could raise the threshold for colonization by potentially pathogenic bacteria thus conferring on the animal 'colonization resistance' (CR). Several antibiotic regimens have evolved, based on this concept (table II), and have been shown to be as effective as the earlier combinations [20, 26, 30, 82]. Drugs which have little effect on the CR include co-trimoxazole, nalidixic acid and polymixin, whereas ampicillin and injectable cephalosporins are likely to suppress the CR. The use of CR-indifferent drugs should reduce the opportunities for the acquisition of antibiotic resistance by the gut flora, and prevent colonization by multi-resistant 'hospital' organisms. In order to achieve the desired results close attention must be paid to the dosages of the oral drugs used and to the choice of antibiotics for treatment of infection.

In recent years, co-trimoxazole has proved to be an effective, better tolerated and inexpensive choice for this purpose [85, 89]. One outcome of co-trimoxazole prophylaxis has been the appearance of colonizing strains of enterobacteria which are not only resistant to the compound, but more alarmingly exhibit multiple antibiotic resistance [91]. The concurrent administration of polymixin B (colistin) may prevent the emergence of co-trimoxazole-resistant enterobacteria [64] and may have the added virtue of inactivating endotoxin in the bowel [3]. A further complication that has been observed with co-trimoxazole prophylaxis in the BMT patient, is myelosuppression causing delay in emergence of the grafted marrow. These deficits may limit the future usefulness of co-trimoxazole. More recently, attention has been paid to the quinolone norfloxacin for this purpose, and the results of detailed studies are awaited.

Few controlled studies have been performed to evaluate antibiotic prophylaxis in BMT recipients, and a protective environment has usually been incorporated into the study arm of the trial [10]. Observations on septicaemia, localised infection and mortality rates, have confirmed the benefits of this combined approach (table III). An additional effect of these measures appears to be a delayed onset and a reduced severity of GVHD [71], and this finding supports the theory that the gut microflora may play a role in the pathogenesis of GVHD [80].

Antifungal Prophylaxis

Antifungals are usually incorporated into the decontamination protocol to suppress yeast overgrowth in the oropharynx and intestine. Traditionally, the polyene antibiotics, amphotericin B and nystatin, have been used either alone or together. The effectiveness of these drugs is not clearly established [44] and as they are not absorbed, systemic prophylaxis is not achieved by their administration. Mepartricin is a haptaene polyene which is absorbed and in a preliminary study has proved as effective as the related polyenes [83]. Ketoconazole, an orally absorbed imidazole, has similarly been compared with amphotericin and nystatin and has also achieved comparable results [28]. In BMT patients two particular problems have emerged with the use of ketoconazole prophylaxis: firstly an interaction with the immunosuppressive drug cyclosporin A which results in elevated and potentially toxic plasma levels of cyclosporin A, probably a result of interference with cellular binding of the drug in the blood [68], and secondly impaired intestinal absorption of ketoconazole believed to be caused by the effects of immunosuppressive agents given before transplant [29]. A further observation in ketoconazole-treated patients has been colonization by resistant *Torulopsis glabrata* [44]. Further studies are therefore necessary before ketoconazole can be recommended for inclusion in prophylactic regimens in BMT patients.

The suppression of skin and mucosal microorganisms with topical antiseptics and antibiotics has been performed with varying degrees of endevour by different transplant units. Chlorhexidine has proved an effective antimicrobial agent [61, 67] and can be used as an aqueous solution for oral and vaginal application and as gel or cream for the gums, teeth and anterior nares. Neomycin has been used for nasal application as a supplement to chlorhexidine and similarly nystatin has been applied to the female lower genital tract for suppression of yeasts. One virtue of these preparations is that they have not been found to promote cross-resistance to drugs that are of value for systemic use.

Antiviral Prophylaxis

Herpes simplex mucositis is the most troublesome early viral complication of BMT, and may occur anytime up to 7 weeks after the start of immunosuppression [48]. The majority of seropositive patients will develop this complication usually involving the oropharynx. Several studies have confirmed the remarkable effectiveness of acyclovir prophylaxis in preventing both reactivation and primary infection when given intravenously [27, 59]. Another study has achieved similar results with oral prophylaxis given between 8 days pre-BMT and 35 days post-BMT [25], and a further interesting observation was the absence of CMV infections throughout the study period in the patients receiving acyclovir; it is clear that these findings require confirmation from other units. Once the drug is stopped the incidence of herpes simplex infection is the same as or higher than for the control group [59]. This phenomenon may paradoxically result from the delay in exposure of the 'new' immune system to the virus due to successful chemoprophylaxis [84]. The isolation of resistant strains of herpes simplex also suggests caution in the widespread prophylactic use of the drug. These strains are mostly mutants which lack the thymidine kinase enzyme essential for converting acyclovir into the active triphosphate form in virus-infected cells [19]. Acyclovir is also effective against varicella-zoster virus and could usefully be given for a longer period after transplant for the prevention of shingles. This could only be practicable with the use of oral preparations, and the results of studies with new analogues of acyclovir which achieve higher serum concentrations after oral administration are eagerly awaited. Unfortunately, acyclovir has no clinically useful direct activity against CMV [49] and alternative strategies for the prevention of CMV pneumonia have had to be adopted. Most interesting so far has been the use of parenteral immunoglobulin or plasma with a high titre of antibody to the virus and the results of three open studies indicate a protective effect [16, 47, 93]. A controlled evaluation is now indicated. Unfortunately, chemoprophylaxis using adenine arabinoside was found not to be effective in preventing CMV pneumonia [40], although the daily dosage used may have been inadequate.

A deficiency of cell-mediated immunity for up to a year after transplant explains the increased occurrence of varicella-zoster infection during this period [18]. The administration of monthly hyperimmune globulin to seronegative recipients may prevent acquisition of the virus or modify the disease, but no study has yet been carried out to answer this question [23].

Protective Isolation

Patients undergoing BMT are normally nursed in a protective environment (PE) in addition to receiving prophylactic antibiotics [10]. No study has yet been undertaken in which a PE was the sole variable under evaluation, but it is rational to protect the neutropenic patient from his 'hostile' environment, both animate and inanimate, and also when at major risk of acquiring airborn infection during intensive treatment for GVH.

The design of PEs varies from the most simple and relatively inexpensive form, a single cubicle with or without filtered air under positive pressure, to laminar flow (LAF) isolators or rooms [42, 54] and plastic isolators or 'bubbles' [79, 90] both of which provide a more stringent barrier to exogenous infection. With air filtration systems particles, including microorganisms, of size greater than 0.3 μm are removed by passage through high efficiency particle arrestor filters. As has been pointed out [1, 96], it would not be possible to manage patients undergoing chemotherapy or BMT if such systems were an absolute requirement. However, pre-fabricated LAF units may offer the most suitable form of protection for the 'high-risk' BMT patient.

Several studies have emanated from the Seattle transplant team which clearly show that exogenous infection can be prevented by combining LAF with prophylactic antibiotics [10, 11, 50] (see table III) and there is the added bonus of modifying GVHD [71]. An integral part of the nursing and medical care of patients in this setting is the use of protective clothing and good handwashing technique by staff, special toilet facilities, 'sterile' water and 'sterile' food [55]. Hospital food has long been recognised as an important source of enterobacteria [56, 60] and the organisation of the dietetics department for the provision of special diets is an important feature of the transplant unit [17].

Indwelling Venous Catheter Care

In recent years the Hickman indwelling right atrial catheter [7, 32] has been widely used to provide ready and continuous access to the circulation during BMT. Local infection and septicaemia are well-known complications observed in patients with catheters in situ [96], occasionally necessitating premature removal and replacement. For prevention of these complications, careful attention is required during insertion of the catheter, which should be carried out by a surgeon experienced in catheter placement using full aseptic technique [77]. Correct positioning of the dacron cuff is important in order to ensure that the catheter is anchored properly in the skin tunnel. Good nursing practice when handling the free end of the catheter, particularly when it is connected to blood-giving sets, has proved effective in reducing the sepsis rate [87].

References

1 Armstrong, D.: Protected environments are discomforting and expensive and do not offer meaningful protection. Am. J. Med. *76:* 685–689 (1984).

2 Atkinson, K.; Storb, R.; Prentice, R.L.; Weiden, P.L.; Witherspoon, R.P.; Sullivan, K.; Noel, D.; Thomas, E.D.: Analysis of late infections in 89 long-term survivors of bone marrow transplantation. Blood *53:* 720–731 (1979).

3 Bannatyne, R.M.; Cheung, R.: Polymixin – an endotoxin inactivator. In Easmon, Gaya, Second international symposium on infections in the immunocompromised host, pp. 279–280 (Academic Press, London 1983).

4 Barrett, A.J.; Kendra, J.R.; Lucas, C.F.; Joss, D.V.; Joshi, R.; Desai, M.; Hugh-Jones, K.; Phillips, R.H.; Rogers, T.R.; Tabara, Z.; Williamson, S.; Hobbs, J.R.: Bone marrow transplantation for acute leukaemia. Br. J. Haemat. *52:* 181–188 (1982).

5 Barrett, A.J.; Kendra, J.R.; Saleem, N.; Desai, S.; Joss, D.V.; Phillips, R.; Rogers, T.R.; Williamson, S.; James, D.C.O.; Hugh-Jones, K.; Hobbs, J.R.: Bone marrow transplantation for acute lymphoblastic leukaemia - the Westminster Hospital experience; in Gale, Recent advances in bone marrow transplantation, pp. 115–122 (Liss, New York 1983).

6 Berkow, R.L.; Weisman, S.J.; Provisor, A.J.; Weetman, R.M.; Baehner, R.L.: Invasive aspergillosis of paranasal tissues in children with malignancies. J. Pediat. *103:* 49–53 (1983).

7 Bjeletich, J.; Hickman, R.O.: The Hickman indwelling catheter. Am. J. Nurs. *80:* 62–65 (1980).

8 Blacklock, H.A.; Pillai, M.V.; Hill, R.S.; Matthews, J.R.D.; Clarke, A.G.; Wade, J.F.: Use of modified subcutaneous right atrial catheter for venous access in leukaemic patients. Lancet *i:* 993–994 (1980).

9 Bodey, G.P.; Buckley, M.; Sathe, Y.S.; Freireich, E.J.: Quantitative relationships between circulating leukocytes and infection in patients with acute leukemia. Ann. intern. Med. *64:* 328–340 (1966).

10 Buckner, C.D.; Clift, R.A.; Sanders, J.E.; Meyers, J.D.; Counts, G.W.; Farewell, V.T.; Thomas, E.D.: Protective environment for marrow transplant recipients. A prospective study. Ann. intern. Med. *89:* 893–901 (1978).

11 Buckner, C.D.; Clift, R.A.; Thomas, E.D.; Hersman, J.; Stewart, P.; Sanders, J.E.: Infection prophylaxis in marrow transplant recipients; in Sasaki, Ozawa, Hashimoto, Recent advances in germfree research, pp. 557–561 (Tokai University Press, Tokyo 1981).

12 Clift, R.A.; Buckner, C.D.: Granulocyte transfusions. Am. J. Med. *76:* 631–636 (1984).

13 Clift, R.A.; Buckner, C.D.; Fefer, A.; Lerner, K.G.; Neiman, P.E.; Storb, R.; Murphy, M.; Thomas, E.D.: Infectious complications of marrow transplantation. Transplant Proc. *6:* 389–393 (1974).

14 Clift, R.A.; Sanders, J.E.; Thomas, E.D.; Williams, B.; Buckner, C.D.: Granulocyte transfusions for the prevention of infection in patients receiving bone-marrow transplants. New Engl. J. Med. *298:* 1052–1057 (1978).

15 Cohen, J.; Donnelly, J.P.; Worsley, A.M.; Catovsky, D.; Goldman, J.M.; Galton, D.A.: Septicaemia caused by viridans streptococci in neutropenic patients with leukaemia. Lancet *ii:* 1452–1454 (1983).

16 Condie, R.M.; O'Reilly, R.J.: Prophylaxis of CMV infection in bone marrow transplant recipients by hyperimmune CMV gammaglobulin. Dev. biol. Stand., vol. 52, pp. 501–513 (Karger, Basel 1982).

17 Cunningham, B.A.; Lenssen, P.; Aker, S.N.; Gittere, K.M.; Cheney, C.L.; Hutchison, M.M.: Nutritional considerations during marrow transplantation. Nurs. Clins N. Am. *18:* 585–596 (1983).

18 Deeg, H.J.; Storb, R.; Thomas, E.D.: Bone marrow transplantation: a review of delayed complications. Br. J. Haemat. *57:* 185–208 (1984).

19 Dekker, C.; Ellis, M.N.; McLaren, C.; Hunter, G.; Rogers, J.; Barry, D.W.: Virus resistance in clinical practice. J. antimicrob. Chemother. *12:* suppl. B, pp. 137–152 (1983).

20 De Vries-Hospers, H.G.; Sleijfer, D.T.; Mulder, N.H.; Waaij, D. van der; Nieweg, H.O.; Saene, H.K.F. van: Infection prevention in patients with acute leukemia by

selective decontamination of the digestive tract (SDD); in Sasaki, Ozawa, Hashimoto, Recent advances in germ-free research, pp. 709–713 (Tokai University Press, Tokyo 1981).
21 Dopfer, R.; Döring, A.; Neithammer, D.: Neutrophil function after allogeneic BMT. Exp. Hematol., Copenh. *11:* suppl. 13, pp. 110–112 (1983).
22 Gale, R.P.; Cline, M.J.; Fahey, J.L.; Feig, S.; Opelz, G.; Young, L.; Territo, M.; Golde, D.; Sparkes, R.; Naeim, N.; Juillard, G.; Haskell, C.; Fawzi, F.; Sarna, G.; Falk, P.: Bone-marrow transplantation in severe aplastic anaemia. Lancet *ii:* 921–923 (1976).
23 Gershon, A.A.: Immunoprophylaxis of varicella-zoster infections. Am. J. Med. *76:* 672–677 (1984).
24 Gerson, S.L.; Talbot, G.H.; Hurwitz, S.; Strom, B.L.; Lusk, E.J.; Cassileth, P.A.: Prolonged granulocytopenia: the major risk factor for invasive pulmonary aspergillosis in patients with acute leukemia. Ann. intern. Med. *100:* 345–351 (1984).
25 Gluckman, E.; Lotsberg, J.; Devergie, A.; Zhao, X.M.; Melo, R.; Gomez-Morales, M.; Nebout, T.; Mazeron, M.C.; Perol, Y.: Prophylaxis of herpes infections after bone-marrow transplantation by oral acyclovir. Lancet *ii:* 706–708 (1983).
26 Guiot, H.F.L.; Van der Meer, J.W.M.; Furth, R. van: Selective antimicrobial modulation of human microbial flora: infection prevention in patients with decreased host defense mechanisms by selective elimination of potentially pathogenic bacteria. J. infect. Dis. *143:* 644–654 (1981).
27 Hann, I.M.; Prentice, H.G.; Blacklock, H.A.; Ross, M.; Brigden, D.; Clark, A.; Burke, C.; Noone, P.; Keaney, M.: Acyclovir prophylaxis of herpes virus infections in severely immunocompromised patients. A randomised double-blind controlled trial. Exp. Hematol., Copenh. *10:* suppl. 10, pp. 2–4 (1982).
28 Hann, I.M.; Prentice, H.G.; Corringham, R.; Blacklock, H.A.; Keaney, M.; Shannon, M.; Noone, P.; Gascoigne, E.; Fox, J.; Boesen, E.; Szawatkowski, M.; Hoffbrand, A.V.: Ketoconazole versus nystatin plus amphotericin B for fungal prophylaxis in severely immunocompromised patients. Lancet *i:* 826–829 (1982).
29 Hann, I.M.; Prentice, H.G.; Keaney, M.; Corringham, R.; Blacklock, A.; Fox, J.; Gascoigne, E.; Van Cutsem, J.: The pharmacokinetics of ketoconazole in severely immunocompromised patients. J. antimicrob. Chemother. *10:* 489–496 (1982).
30 Henry, S.A.: Chemoprophylaxis of bacterial infections in granulocytopenic patients. Am. J. Med. *76:* 645–651 (1984).
31 Henslee, J.; Bostrum, B.; Weisdorf, D.; Ramsay, N.; McGlave, P.; Kersey, J.: Streptococcal sepsis in bone marrow transplant patients. Lancet *i:* 393 (1984).
32 Hickman, R.O.; Buckner, C.D.; Clift, R.A.; Sanders, J.E.; Stewart, P.; Thomas, E.D.: A modified right atrial catheter for access to the venous system in marrow transplant recipients. Surg. Obstet. Gynec. *148:* 871–875 (1979).
33 Hobbs, J.R.: Bone marrow transplantation for inborn errors. Lancet *ii:* 735–739 (1981).
34 Hughes, W.T.; Kuhn, S.; Chaudhary, S.; Feldman, S.; Verzosa, M.; Rhomes, J.A.; Aur, M.D.; Pratt, C.; George, S.L.: Successful chemoprophylaxis for *Pneumocystis carinii* pneumonitis. New Engl. J. Med. *297:* 1419–1426 (1977).
35 Johnson, F.L.; Hartmann, J.R.; Thomas, E.D.; Chard, R.L.; Hersman, J.A.;

Buckner, C.D.; Clift, R.A.; Storb, R.: Marrow transplantation in treatment of children with aplastic anaemia or acute leukaemia. Archs Dis. Childh. *51:* 403–410 (1976).
36 Joss, D.V.; Desai, S.; Bannerjee, G.; Ingram, L.; Hugh-Jones, K.; Barrett, A.J.; Hobbs, J.R.: Alterations in xylose absorption and its relationship to cyclosporin A conditioning regimes and gut pathology after bone marrow transplantation. Exp. Hematol., Copenh. *11:* supp. 13, pp. 34–36 (1983).
37 Kendra, J.R.; Barrett, A.J.; Lucas, C.; Joshi, R.; Joss, V.; Desai, M.; Halil, O.; Rogers, T.R.; Hobbs, J.R.; Hugh-Jones, K.: Response of graft versus host disease to high doses of methylprednisolone. Clin. Lab. Haemat. *3:* 19–26 (1981).
38 Kendra, J.R.; Lucas, C.F.; Chambers, D.; Williamson, S.; Byrom, N.; Foroozanfar, N.; Joss, D.V.; Horsler, H.; James, D.C.O.; Selwyn, S.; Rogers, T.R.; Henry, K.; Phillips, R.H.; Barrett, A.J.; Hugh-Jones, K.; Hobbs, J.R.: Bone marrow transplantation for severe aplastic anaemia a review of the Westminster experience of 24 cases. Clin. Lab. Haemat. *5:* 131–143 (1983).
39 King, A.; Rampling, A.; Wight, D.G.D.; Warren, R.E.: Neutropenic enterocolitis due to *Clostridium septicum* infection. J. clin. Path. *37:* 335–343 (1984).
40 Kraemer, K.G.; Neiman, P.E.; Reeves, W.C.; Thomas, E.D.: Prophylactic adenine arabinoside following marrow transplantation. Transplant. Proc. *10:* 237–240 (1978).
41 Levine, A.S.; Siegel, S.E.; Schreiber, A.D.; Hauser, J.; Preisler, H.; Goldstein, I.M.; Seidler, F.; Simon, R.; Perry, S.; Bennett, J.E.; Henderson, E.S.: Protected environments and prophylactic antibiotics. New Engl. J. Med. *288:* 477–483 (1973).
42 Lindgren, P.S.: The laminar air flow room: nursing practices and procedures. Nurs. Clins N. Am. *18:* 553–561 (1983).
43 Mathé, G.; Schwarzenberg, L.: Bone-marrow transplantation in France, 1958–1973. Transplant. Proc. *6:* 335–343 (1974).
44 Meunier-Carpentier, F.: Chemoprophylaxis of fungal infections. Am. J. Med. *76:* 652–656 (1984).
45 Meyers, J.D.; Atkinson, K.: Infection in bone marrow transplantation; in Nathan, Clinics in haematology, vol. 12, pp. 791–811 (Saunders, London 1983).
46 Meyers, J.D.; Fluornoy, N.; Thomas, E.D.: Cytomegalovirus infection and specific cell-mediated immunity after marrow transplant. J. infect. Dis. *142:* 816–824 (1980).
47 Meyers, J.D.; Leszczynski, J.; Zaia, J.A.; Flournoy, N.; Newton, B.; Snydman, D.R.; Wright, G.G.; Levin, M.J.; Thomas, E.D.: Prevention of cytomegalovirus infection by cytomegalovirus immuneglobulin after marrow transplantation. Ann. intern. Med. *98:* 442–446 (1983).
48 Meyers, J.D.; Thomas, E.D.: Infection complicating bone marrow transplantation; in Rubin, Young, Clinical approach to infection in the compromised host., pp. 507–551 (Plenum, Press, New York 1981).
49 Meyers, J.D.; Wade, J.C.; McGuffin, R.W.; Springmeyer, S.C.; Thomas, E.D.: The use of acyclovir for cytomegalovirus infections in the immunocompromised host. J. antimicrob. Chemother. *12:* suppl. B, pp. 181–193 (1983).
50 Navari, R.M.; Buckner, C.D.; Clift, R.A.; Storb, R.; Sanders, J.E.; Stewart, P.; Sullivan, K.M.; Williams, B.; Counts, G.W.; Meyers, J.D.; Thomas, E.D.: Prophylaxis of infection in patients with aplastic anaemia receiving allogeneic marrow transplants. Am. J. Med. *76:* 564–572 (1984).

51 Neiman, P.E.; Reeves, W.; Ray, G.; Fluornoy, N.; Lerner, K.G.; Sale, G.E.; Thomas, E.D.: A prospective analysis of interstitial pneumonia and opportunistic viral infection among recipients of allogeneic bone marrow grafts. J. infect. Dis. *136:* 754–767 (1977).

52 Neiman, P.; Wasserman, P.B.; Wentworth, B.B.; Kao, G.F.; Lerner, K.G.; Storb, R.; Buckner, C.D.; Clift, R.A.; Fefer, A.; Fass, L.; Glucksberg, H.; Thomas, E.D.: Interstitial pneumonia and cytomegalovirus infection as complications of human marrow transplantation. Transplantation *15:* 478–485 (1973).

53 O'Reilly, R.J.; Lee, F.K.; Grossbard, E.; Kapoor, N.; Kirkpatrick, D.; Dinsmore, R.; Stutzer, C.; Shah, K.V.; Nahmias, A.J.: Papovavirus excretion following marrow transplantation: incidence and association with hepatic dysfunction. Transplant. Proc. *13:* 262–266 (1981).

54 Penland, W.Z.; Perry, S.: Portable laminar-air-flow isolator. Lancet *i:* 174–176 (1970).

55 Pizzo, P.A.: How to prevent the acquisition of potential pathogens; in Spitzy, Karrer, Proceedings of 13th International Congress of Chemotherapy, part 3, pp. 15–21 (Egermann, Vienna 1983).

56 Pizzo, P.A.; Purvis, D.S.; Waters, C.: Microbiological evaluation of food items for patients undergoing gastrointestinal decontamination and protected isolation. J. Am. diet. Ass. *81:* 272–279 (1982).

57 Pizzo, P.A.; Robichaud, K.J.; Wesley, R.; Commers, J.R.: Fever in the pediatric and young adult patient with cancer. A prospective study of 1001 episodes. Medicine *61:* 153–165 (1982).

58 Powles, R.L.; Morgenstern, G.R.; Clink, H.M.; Hedley, D.; Bandini, G.; Lumley, H.; Watson, J.G.; Lawson, D.; Spence, D.; Barrett, A.; Jameson, B.; Lawler, S.; Kay, H.E.M.; McElwain, T.J.: The place of bone marrow transplantation in acute myelogenous leukaemia. Lancet *i:* 1047–1050 (1980).

59 Prentice, H.G.: Use of acyclovir for prophylaxis of herpes infections in severely immunocompromised patients. J. antimicrob. Chemother. *12:* suppl. B, pp. 153–159 (1983).

60 Remington, J.S.; Schimpff, S.C.: Please don't eat the salads. New Engl. J. Med. *304:* 433–435 (1981).

61 Rogers, T.R.; Hall, G.; Anderson, I.S.; Smith, N.R.; Selwyn, S.: Factors influencing microbial attachment to buccal epithelial cells in immunodeficient patients; in Sasaki, Ozawa, Hashimoto, Recent advances in germfree research, pp. 173–177 (Tokai University Press, Tokyo 1981).

62 Rogers, T.R.; Petrou, M.; Lucas, C.; Chung, J.T.N.; Barrett, A.J.; Borriello, S.P.; Honour, P.: Spread of *Clostridium difficile* among patients receiving non-absorbable antibiotics for gut decontamination. Br. med. J. *283:* 408–409 (1981).

63 Rogers, T.R.; White, S.; Pallett, A.; Lucas, C.; Tabara, Z.: An investigation into the relationship between *Staphylococcus epidermidis* bacteremia and the use of Hickman catheters during marrow transplantation. Exp. Hematol., Copenh. *10:* suppl. 10, p. 12 (1982).

64 Rozenberg-Arska, M.; Dekker, A.W.; Verhoef, J.: The effect of addition of colistin to the trimethoprim/sulphamethoxazole (TMP/SMZ) regimen for prevention of infection in patients with acute non-lymphocytic leukaemia; in Easmon, Gaya, Second International Symposium on Infections in the Immunocompromised Host, pp. 265–267 (Academic Press, London 1983).

65 Santos, G.: History of bone marrow transplantation; in Nathan, Clinics in haematology, No. 12, pp. 611–639 (Saunders, London 1983).
66 Schimpff, S.C.: Infection prevention during profound granulocytopenia. Ann. intern. Med. *93:* 358–361 (1980).
67 Selwyn, S.; Anderson, I.S.; Rogers, T.R.: Quantitative studies on the decontamination of skin and mucous membranes in relation to immunodeficient patients; in Fliedner, Heit, Niethammer, Pflieger, Clinical and experimental gnotobiotics. Zentbl. Bakt. ParasitKde, suppl. 7, pp. 281–284 (Fischer, Stuttgart 1979).
68 Smith, J.; Hows, J.; Donnelly, P.; Baughan, A.; Goldman, J.; Gordon-Smith, E.C.: Interaction of cyclosporin A and ketoconazole. Exp. Hematol., Copenh. *11:* suppl. 13, pp. 176–178 (1983).
69 Solberg, C.O.; Meuwissen, H.J.; Needham, R.N.; Good, R.A.; Matsen, J.M.: Infectious complications in bone marrow transplant patients. Br. med. J. *i:* 18–23 (1971).
70 Stamm, W.E.; Tompkins, L.S.; Wagner, K.F.; Counts, G.W.; Thomas, E.D.; Meyers, J.D.: Infection due to *Corynebacterium* species in marrow transplant patients. Ann. intern. Med. *91:* 167–173 (1979).
71 Storb, R.; Prentice, R.L.; Buckner, C.D.; Clift, R.A.; Appelbaum, F.J.; Sullivan, K.M.; Witherspoon, R.P.; Thomas, E.D.: Graft-versus-host disease and survival in patients with aplastic anemia treated by marrow grafts from HLA-identical siblings. Beneficial effect of a protective environment. New Engl. J. Med. *308:* 302–307 (1983).
72 Storring, R.A.; Jameson, B.; McElwain, T.J.; Wiltshaw, E.; Spiers, A.S.D.; Gaya, H.: Oral non-absorbed antibiotics prevent infection in acute non-lymphoblastic leukaemia. Lancet *ii:* 837–840 (1977).
73 Strauss, R.G.: Therapeutic neutrophil transfusions: are controlled studies no longer appropriate? Am. J. Med. *65:* 1001–1006 (1978).
74 Ten Napel, C.H.H.; The, T.H.: Acute cytomegalovirus infection and the host immune response. II Relationship of suppressed in vitro lymphocyte reactivity to bacterial recall antigens and mitogens with the development of cytomegalovirus-induced lymphocyte reactivity. Clin. exp. Immunol. *39:* 272–278 (1980).
75 Thomas, E.D.; Buckner, C.D.; Banaji, M.; Clift, R.A.; Fefer, A.; Fluornoy, N.; Goodelz, B.W.; Hickman, R.O.; Lerner, K.G.; Neiman, P.E.; Sale, G.E.; Sanders, J.E.; Singer, J.; Stevens, M.; Storb, R.; Weiden, P.L.: One hundred patients with acute leukaemia treated by chemotherapy, total body irradiation, and allogeneic marrow transplantation. Blood *49:* 511–553 (1977).
76 Thomas, E.D.; Storb, R.; Clift, R.A.; Fefer, A.; Johnson, F.L.; Neiman, P.E.; Lerner, K.G.; Glucksberg, H.; Buckner, C.D.: Bone-marrow transplantation (First of two parts). New Engl. J. Med. *292:* 832–843 (1975).
77 Thomas, M.: The use of the Hickman catheter in the management of patients with leukaemia and other malignancies. Br. J. Surg. *66:* 673–674 (1979).
78 Townsend, T.R.; Bolyard, E.A.; Yolken, R.H.; Beschorner, W.E.; Bishop, C.A.; Burns, W.H.; Santos, G.W.; Saral, R.: Outbreak of coxsackie A1 gastroenteritis. A complication of bone marrow transplantation. Lancet *i:* 820–823 (1982).
79 Trexler, P.C.; Spiers, A.S.D.; Gaya, H.: Plastic isolators for treatment of acute leukaemia patients under "germ-free" conditions. Br. med. J. *iv:* 549–552 (1975).
80 Truitt, R.L.; Bortin, M.M.; Rimm, A.A.: Successful adoptive immunotherapy of AKR spontaneous T cell leukaemia following antibiotic decontamination and pro-

tective isolation; in Fliedner, Heit, Niethammer, Pflieger, Clinical and experimental gnotobiotics. Zentbl. Bakt. ParasitKde, suppl. 7, pp. 215–220 (Fischer, Stuttgart 1979).

81 Van der Waaij, D.; Berghuis, J.M.; Lekkerkerk, J.E.C.: Colonization resistance of the digestive tract of mice during systemic antibiotic treatment. J. Hyg., Camb. *70:* 605–610 (1972).

82 Van der Waaij, D.: Colonization resistance; in Easmon, Gaya, Second international symposium on infections in the immunocompromised host, pp. 55–60 (Academic Press, London 1983).

83 Van Lint, M.T.; Bacigalupo, A.; Frassoni, F.; Podesta, M.; Soro, O.; Pedulla, D.; Marmont, A.M.: Ketoconazole versus mepartricin for the prevention of candida infections in the immunocompromized host. Exp. Hematol., Copenh. *10:* suppl. 10, pp. 6–7 (1982).

84 Wade, J.C.; Newton, B.; McLaren, C.; Flournoy, N.; Kelney, R.E.; Meyers, J.D.: Intravenous acyclovir to treat mucocutaneous herpes simplex virus infection after marrow transplantation. A double-blind trial. Ann. intern. Med. *96:* 265–269 (1982).

85 Wade, J.C.; Schimpff, S.C.; Hargadon, M.T.; Fortner, C.L.; Young, V.M.; Weirnik, P.H.: A comparison of tremethoprim-sulfamethoxazole plus nystatin with gentamicin plus nystatin in the prevention of infections in acute leukemia. New Engl. J. Med. *304:* 1057–1062 (1981).

86 Wade, J.C.; Schimpff, S.C.; Newman, K.A.; Wiernik, P.H.: Staphylococcus epidermidis. An increasing cause of infection in patients with granulocytopenia. Ann. intern. Med. *97:* 503–508 (1982).

87 Watson, A.J.: Preventing infection from Hickman lines. Nursing Times May 11th, pp. 25–26 (1983).

88 Watson, J.G.: Problems of infection after bone marrow transplantation. J. clin. Path. *36:* 683–692 (1983).

89 Watson, J.G.; Jameson, B.; Powles, R.L.; McElwain, T.J.; Lawson, D.N.; Judson, I.; Morgenstern, G.R.; Lumley, H.; Kay, H.E.M.: Co-trimoxazole versus non-absorbable antibiotics in acute leukaemia. Lancet *i:* 6–9 (1982).

90 Watson, J.G.; Rogers, T.R.; Selwyn, S.; Smith, R.G.: Evaluation of Vickers-Trexler isolator in children undergoing bone marrow transplantation. Archs Dis. Childh. *52:* 563–568 (1977).

91 Wilson, J.M.; Guiney, D.G.: Failure of oral trimethoprim-sulfamethoxazole prophylaxis in acute leukemia. Isolation of resistant plasmids from strains of enterobacteriaciae causing bacteremia. New Engl. J. Med. *306:* 16–20 (1982).

92 Winston, D.J.; Gale, R.P.; Meyer, D.V.; Young, L.S.; UCLA Bone Marrow Transplantation Group: Infectious complications of human bone marrow transplantation. Medicine *58:* 1–31 (1979).

93 Winston, D.J.; Pollard, R.B.; Ho, W.G.; Gallagher, J.G.; Rasmussen, L.E.; Nan-Ying, S.; Lin, C.H.; Gossett, T.G.; Merigan, T.C.; Gale, R.P.: Cytomegalovirus immune plasma in bone marrow transplant recipients. Ann. intern. Med. *97:* 11–18 (1982).

94 Yolken, R.H.; Bishop, C.A.; Townsend, T.R.; Bolyard, E.A.; Bartlett, J.; Santos, G.W.; Saral, R.: Infectious gastroenteritis in bone-marrow-transplant recipients. New Engl. J. Med. *306:* 1009–1012 (1982).

95 Young, L.S.: Management of infections in leukemia and lymphoma; Rubin, Young, Clinical approach to infection in the compromised host, pp. 461-506 (Plenum, Press, New York 1981).
96 Zaia, J.A.: Infections; in Blume, Petz, Clinical bone marrow transplantation, pp. 131-176 (Churchill-Livingstone, New York 1983).

T.R. Rogers, MSc, MRCPath, Department of Medical Microbiology, Westminster Medical School, Horseferry Road, London SW1P 2AR (UK)

Antibiot. Chemother., vol. 33, pp. 114–139 (Karger, Basel 1985)

Perioperative Prevention of Infection in Cardiac Surgery

Thomas R. Beam, Jr.

Buffalo VA Medical Center, State University of New York at Buffalo, Buffalo, N.Y., USA

Introduction

Prevention of infection in open-heart surgery has been a primary objective of every physician involved in the care of patients undergoing the surgical procedures classified in this category. Published literature has focused on prosthetic valve and coronary artery bypass graft procedures. It is clear that much of the framework for infection prevention and control developed in the 1960s and early 1970s. Recent observations justify modification of some of these previously established principles.

In this chapter I will review the epidemiology of postoperative infectious complications of open-heart surgery; identify the pathogens responsible for these infections; explain the rationale for preventive measures applied to the environment, operating room (OR) personnel and the patient; appraise the information available about various antibiotics used as prophylactic agents; discuss the duration of antimicrobial prophylaxis, and conclude with an assessment of current practices and the economic impact of prophylaxis options available to the physician.

Epidemiology of Perioperative Infections in Cardiac Surgery

There are three potential sources of contamination during open heart surgery: (1) the environment; (2) OR personnel; (3) the patient. Each has been studied for relevance to postoperative infectious complications.

Environmental Contamination

The OR and its ventilation system can serve as a focus for infectious particles. One of the best examples is contamination by *Aspergillus* spp. [1]. Organisms capable of surviving in spore form can remain viable in the inanimate environment and be a cause of postoperative infection. Use of HEPA filters can substantially reduce this form of contamination [2]. Periodic cleaning of surfaces (i.e., floors, walls, ceilings) along with ventilation covers and shafts can reduce contamination to essentially zero.

Proving that postoperative bacterial infections result from high levels of airborne contamination has been much more difficult [3]. Most often the bacteria collected on settling plates originate from people in the OR. Correlation of the types of bacteria isolated with subsequent wound infections almost never occurs [4]. However, studies conducted in orthopedic surgery with lengthy operative time and a large exposed wound support the contention that a clean environment should be advantageous to clean surgery [5]. Therefore, use of HEPA filters, high air exchange rates and periodic cleaning are endorsed. Laminar flow is expensive and not proven to be necessary to minimize infectious complications in open-heart surgery.

There are numerous opportunities for bacterial contamination of intraoperative devices. Arterial pressure devices, central venous lines, Swan-Ganz catheters and peripheral intravenous catheters are all routinely employed. Each is associated with a small but definite risk for producing contamination [6]. Of greater importance is the duration these devices remain in place. *Maki* [7] has proven that risk increases exponentially as time proceeds linearly. Pressure transducers and domes can also be the focus for postoperative septic complications [8].

Anesthesia equipment or respirators can be contaminated and produce postoperative pneumonic complications. The use of disposable supplies and careful monitoring of water sources have eliminated this potential hazard from serious consideration [9]. Suction devices may also become contaminated, especially with water-borne organisms such as *Pseudomonas* [10]. Severe sternotomy wound infections have resulted.

All studies of extracorporeal circulation devices have shown that bacterial contamination is the rule rather than the exception [9]. Moreover, the yield of positive cultures can be substantially increased by inactivating the prophylactic antibiotics administered for the procedure

[11]. Despite these findings there has rarely been a significant correlation between isolates obtained from bypass equipment and postoperative infectious complications.

Blakemore et al. [4] felt that OR personnel contributed a large pool of organisms to the air. These bacteria then contaminated the suction lines and ultimately the patient's blood. Factors responsible for the virulence of certain strains were not identified. This postulate may occasionally be correct, but the organisms causing infection are most often different from those contaminating the extracorporeal circulation device.

In patients with marginal cardiac output, the intra-aortic balloon pump (IABP) is often used. It is placed under sterile conditions but may be left in place for several postoperative days. There have been no published studies evaluating the risk of infection or prophylaxis against infection when the IABP is used. A newly developed percutaneous IABP eliminates the need for vascular cutdown and potentially reduces the risk of infectious complications. But the normal cutaneous barrier is violated, and device-related infections are still a cause for concern.

Cardioplegic solutions can be contaminated, particularly if ice is used to cool them. Similarly, intravenous fluids [12] and transfusates can serve as a rare source of contamination. Some operations require the use of cryoprecipitate. *Pseudomonas cepacia* has been isolated from the ports of cryoprecipitate bags [13].

One final contaminant is directly related to the use of bioprosthetic materials in open-heart surgery. Porcine valves may be infected with *Mycobacterium chelonei.* A postoperative endocarditis results [14]. Mycobacteria also have been identified as occasional environmental contaminants [15] and can best be removed by ultrafiltration of air and surface cleaning.

Several groups have described efforts to reduce postoperative infectious complications by modifying the environment. But multiple potential sources of contamination have been changed simultaneously. It thus is impossible to determine which measure or measures may be critical in lessening risk to the patient. Studies were also conducted sequentially rather than with concurrent controls. This further compromises interpretation of the results. For example, *Hughes* [16] reported unacceptably high risk of endocarditis at the Wadsworth VA Medical Center. Changes implemented included: (1) use of systemic antimicrobial prophylaxis; (2) application of topical antibiotic ointment on the nares of carriers of 'pathogens'; (3) resolution of all dental problems; (4) use of clean, private rooms preoperatively; (5) sterilized laundry; (6) restriction of patient movement; (7) hexachlorophene bathing thrice daily for 5 days; (8) preoperative cleaning of the OR; (9) use of positive pressure in the OR compared to outside hallways; (10) reducing the number of personnel moving through the room; (11) improved oxygenator and heat exchanger equipment; (12) conversion from reusable glass to disposable plastic syringes; (13) filtration of oxygen sources; (14) change of suture material; (15) use of plastic sheets in place of towels to reduce wicking; (16) altered procedures for sterilizing the bypass pump; and (17) soaking of prosthetic valves in antibiotic solution. After instituting these changes, 0 of 86 subsequent patients developed prosthetic-valve endocarditis (PVE) [16].

A similarly complex project was reported by *Clark* et al. [17]. Changes included renovation of the OR, installation of a high-flow HEPA-filtered vertical ventilation system, change in gowns and drapes to less permeable materials, steam sterilization of prosthetic valves, use of antistaphylococcal antibiotic prophylaxis, and unannounced bacteriologic surveillance of OR personnel. Deep wound infections were reduced from 2.9 to 0.6%, a statistically significant change. Which of the measure(s) proved important to the reduction of infectious complications is unknown.

Personnel

Extensive studies have been conducted to evaluate the possible role of OR personnel contaminating the patient's wound. The best epidemiologic studies have traced staphylococci. Correlation of antibiogram and phage-typing yields a high likelihood that the transmission of a strain can be accurately followed.

Staphylococci may colonize the anterior nares in as many as 40% of hospitalized patients and 70% of hospital staff. During times of high rates of staphylococcal infections, these numbers may increase substantially. Most people carry the organism and do not shed it into the surrounding environment. Intercurrent respiratory illnesses may convert a carrier to a shedder, but often there is no identifiable factor which precipitates this change [18].

Bernard and Cole [19] evaluated personnel at Barnes Hospital and Washington University. They determined that 20% of all gloves developed punctures during surgery. 4,000–18,000 organisms could be shed into a wound through a broken glove in 20 min by a carrier of staphylococci despite adequate surgical scrub of the hands. Moreover, when the surgeon's skin came in contact with blood or serum, there was a rapid increase in the number of bacteria shed.

Despite the fact that 100% of surgeons participating in this study carried staphylococci, patients were most often the source of their own infection. Of 100 consecutive patients undergoing abdominal operations, 14 carried staphylococci preoperatively and 7 continued to carry the same organism postoperatively. 4 developed postoperative staphylococcal wound infections, all caused by the same phage type they carried. Neither phage types carried by the surgeons nor those isolated from the environment played a role in wound infections.

Burke [20] conducted a similar study among patients undergoing either thoracic or abdominal procedures but added a saline lavage culture obtained from the surgical wound prior to closure. Coagulase-positive staphylococci were isolated from 92% of the cases. The number of organisms increased proportionately to the duration of the surgical procedure. But only 3 of the 50 wounds contained phage types carried by OR personnel. 1 of the 2 wound infections which followed surgery could be traced to the patient's own flora. The source of the second infection was not found.

Howe and Marston [21] performed cultures of patients, personnel and the inanimate environment. They were not so successful in identifying the source of staphylococcal infections as were the previously cited authors. But they did find that only 3 strains among 15 patient infections from 282 procedures correlated with phage types carried by personnel. *Meleney* [22], in evaluating streptococcal wound infections, reached a similar conclusion. That is, the strain producing a postoperative wound infection was more likely to originate from the patient than from hospital personnel.

During the course of a comparative evaluation of cefoperazone and cephalothin prophylaxis in coronary artery bypass graft surgery, we encountered an outbreak of staphylococcal infections [23]. *Staphylococcus aureus,* phage type 96, was isolated from a donor site infection in January, 1981. 4 subsequent infections were caused by this strain, equally divided between cephalothin and cefoperazone prophylaxis. Phage type 96 staphylococci were not isolated from any of the patients preoperatively. One surgeon carried this strain in the anterior nares. All environmental cultures were negative for staphylococci.

Cardiothoracic surgical procedures were discontinued until 1 week of topical neomycin/polymixin ointment had been used and the strain was eradicated from the surgeon-carrier. Subsequent patients were not infected by phage type 96 staphylococci. However, the surgeon became colonized with a new phage type, and one postoperative infection was caused by this strain. At no time during this outbreak of infections did the surgeon have an upper respiratory tract infection. The reason for his shedding of staphylococci remains unknown. The experience, though dramatic and critically important, remains the exception rather than the rule. Most infections result from the patient's endogenous flora and not from hospital personnel.

Patients

As noted in the previous section, the patient (and his or her endogenous bacterial flora) is the most common source of bacteria which result in postoperative wound infections. There are several additional risk factors related to the patient's health status which predispose to infectious complications. *Simchen* et al. [24] have defined these factors in a prospective evaluation of 372 patients undergoing cardiac surgery. This study, as well as others [25, 26], showed that reoperation during the same admission was associated with excessive risk of infectious complications. Duration of surgery beyond 6 h, operations performed on patients age 65 years or older, and functional cardiac status assessed preoperatively each served as an independent risk factor for increased infection rate.

Ehrenkranz [27] evaluated 9,108 clean surgical procedures performed in community hospitals. Remote infection at the time of surgery, diabetes mellitus and operations lasting longer than 4 h were important variables in subsequent infectious complications. Additional risk factors in clean surgical procedures include obesity and steroid therapy [28].

In conclusion, the patient undergoing open-heart surgery is at risk for postoperative infectious complications. The most likely source of contaminating organisms is the patient himself. Meticulous attention should be paid to personnel practices, especially aseptic technique. Maintaining a clean environment is also important, but the inanimate

Table I. Bacterial etiology of early PVE

Authors	Reference	Period reviewed	Number of cases		Organism, number of cases		
			total	early PVE	*S. aureus*	*S. epidermidis*	gram-negative bacilli
Amoury et al.	86	1956–1965	357	13	1	11	2
Stein et al.	87	–1965[1]	288	15	11[2]	1	4[2]
Dismukes et al.	88	1964–1971	1,671	19	2	3	2
Slaughter et al.	89	1960–1972	1,236	23	5	8	4
Wilson et al.	90	1963–1974	4,586	16	7	1	6
Aintablian et al.	91	1971–1974	234	3	0	2	1
Rossiter et al.	92	1963–1977	2,184	9	2	3	0
Masur and Johnson	93	1962–1978	1,282	16	1	8	0

[1] First year of study not stated.
[2] 2 cases with polymicrobial isolates.

environment is the least likely contributor to nosocomial infections in cardiac surgery patients.

Bacteria responsible for Postoperative Infections in Open-Heart Surgery

Meleney's [22] work demonstrated that streptococci were a major postoperative concern in clean surgery performed during the preantibiotic era. From the epidemiologic studies conducted in the 1960s it is apparent that *S. aureus* was the most common pathogen responsible for postoperative infection. These observations parallel the changes noted in etiologic agents of nosocomial infections in general [29]. In the 1970s, gram-negative enteric bacteria assumed the preeminent role in nosocomial infections [30]. But there has not been a dramatic increase in the incidence of gram-negative bacillary PVE, as shown in table I.

Delgado and Cobbs [31] tabulated results from several large series of patients undergoing implantation of valvular prostheses at medical centers in the United States. Early prosthetic valve endocarditis (occurring within 2 months of surgery), is most often caused by staphylococci. *Staphylococcus epidermidis* is more commonly isolated than *S. aureus.* Rates of infection usually range from 0.5 to 1.0%. Postoperative wound infections can cause major morbidity and mortality. But concern is directed toward prevention of PVE, since infection often mandates valve replacement. Table I shows that the etiology of early PVE has remained stable for the past 20 years.

S. epidermidis and *S. aureus* continue to be important pathogens because of the presence of prosthetic material. Recent studies with *S. epidermidis* have shown that this organism produces slime which may serve as a barrier to the action of both antibiotics and host defenses [32]. The bacteria are also capable of eroding the surface of polyethylene, allowing quantitatively minor intraoperative contamination to attain major clinical significance [33].

Further concern must be expressed over the increasing prevalence of resistance to methicillin and first-generation cephalosporins among staphylococci [34]. If patients become colonized with methicillin-resistant *S. aureus* or *S. epidermidis* preoperatively, then the number of cases of PVE caused by methicillin-resistant staphylococci should also increase in the next few years. Because methicillin-resistant staphylococci have been identified in all types of hospitals in the United States and not just university referral centers [35], this possibility seems likely to occur.

Gram-negative bacilli as a group form the second most common etiologic agents of PVE. Of 178 patients in the series of *Delgado and Cobbs* [31] 22% were infected by these bacteria. They were assumed to contaminate the site directly during surgery or subsequently during transient bacteremia. Complications such as paravalvular leak and embolic phenomena are seen with these organisms at a frequency similar to that observed with gram-positive infections. Combined surgical and medical therapy maximizes the chance of successful patient outcome.

In coronary artery bypass graft procedures, autologous saphenous veins or the internal mammary artery serve as the most frequent donor material. The gravest form of infectious postoperative complication is mediastinitis with concurrent bacteremia. But postoperative donor site infections are also important and cause excess morbidity and extended hospital stay [36].

The incidence and etiology of postoperative mediastinitis are presented in table II. The earlier series of *Bain* et al. [37] and *Sutherland* et

Table II. Bacterial etiology of postoperative mediastinitis in coronary artery bypass graft surgery

Authors	Reference	Period reviewed	Number of cases		Organism, number of cases		
			total	mediastinitis	*S. aureus*	*S. epidermidis*	gram-negative bacilli
Sanfelippo and Danielson	94	-1972[1]	27	12	1	2	8
Engelman et al.	95	1970–1972	360	9	0	5[2]	5[2]
Culliford et al.	96	1971–1974	956	20	not stated	not stated	not stated
Bain et al.	37	1976	100	5	4	0	1
Stoney et al.	97	1970–1977	4,077	20	2	8	10
Sutherland et al.	38	1976–1979	693	6	6	0	0
Bor et al.	98	1975–1979	349 (616)[3]	7 (21)	(5)	(6)	(11)
Wells et al.	39	not stated	175	12	3[4]	0	11[4]

[1] First year of study not stated.
[2] 4 patients had multiple isolates.
[3] Numbers in parentheses indicate data for total series; specific rates for coronary artery bypass procedures cannot be discerned.
[4] Some patients had multiple isolates.

al. [38] demonstrated that *S. aureus* is an important postoperative pathogen. But the more recent report of *Wells* et al. [39] clearly documents the importance of gram-negative bacilli in postoperative wound infections. The majority of both mediastinal and donor site infections were caused by gram-negative enteric organisms. Strains included *Klebsiella, Acinetobacter, Citrobacter, Proteus* and *Escherichia coli*. These findings were confirmed by *Farrington* et al. [40], who speculate that the chest wound infections may be caused by contaminated donor vein grafts. Wound infections at both sites are caused by similar bacterial flora.

Alternatively, patients are hospitalized long enough to acquire nosocomial flora. These newly acquired strains may then serve as the reservoir for autoinfection [29]. At the Buffalo VA Medical Center patients are hospitalized an average of 4 days preoperatively. This is sufficient time to acquire and carry nosocomial strains [41].

A third possibility is that the patients are carriers of gram-negative enteric bacilli prior to hospitalization. Factors likely to increase the probability of carrying gram-negative bacilli include age, underlying diseases, level of prehospital institutionalization, recent prior hospitalization, and recent use of antibiotics [42]. Patients undergoing coronary artery bypass graft procedures clearly have several of these risk factors. We found our patients had a mean age of 58.4 years and 1.8 underlying diseases in one previous study [43], and a mean age of 58.5 years and 1.3 underlying diseases in a more recent study [44]. Carriage of gram-negative bacilli upon entry to the hospital was not assessed. Tracing the epidemiology of postoperative wound infections caused by gram-negative bacilli will be much more difficult than following staphylococci, unless a multiple antibiotic-resistant strain is responsible for postoperative infections [45], DNA fingerprinting [46], or serotyping [47] is performed.

Serious bacterial infections continue to occur in open-heart surgery. During of the implantation of foreign materials, *S. aureus* and *S. epidermidis* must remain of foremost concern. Prophylactic measures must focus on the characteristics and epidemiology of these organisms. Gram-negative bacilli are a second but lesser concern. In coronary artery bypass graft surgery many studies have proven that staphylococci cannot be ignored. But gram-negative rods have emerged as the major pathogens in postoperative wound infections. Preventive measures must be directed toward these organisms and may differ somewhat from modalities employed in valvular surgery.

Antibiotics for Prophylaxis against Infection in Open-Heart Surgery

The rate of postoperative infections is generally considered to be low. The procedures are defined as clean rather than clean-contaminated, since no mucosal surface is transected. Therefore, the need for prophylactic antibiotics has been argued.

The rationale for prophylaxis is derived from the early studies of *Miles* et al. [48], *Burke* [49], and *Dineen* [50, 51]. In brief, these investigators created surgical incisions on the abdominal wall of guinea pigs. A standardized inoculum of several different strains of bacteria was applied. Antimicrobial prophylaxis was administered prior to, simultaneous with, shortly after or markedly after contamination of the wound.

A critical interval of microbial susceptibility was defined. Antibiotics needed to be delivered just prior to inoculation or within 3 h of that time. Late administration of drugs afforded no benefit over controls [49].

Furthermore, the in vitro susceptibility of a bacterial strain served as a predictor of prophylactic efficacy. So long as tissue concentrations of antibiotic exceeded the minimum inhibitory concentration (MIC), host defenses could control and remove the bacterial inoculum. Expressed in different terms, a bacteriostatic antibiotic could be successfully employed as a prophylactic agent (erythromycin in experimental staphylococcal infection). Eradication did not depend solely on antibiotic killing activity. In addition, effective antimicrobial prophylaxis could be rendered inadequate by manipulating host defenses [48].

Need for Prophylactic Antibiotics

If the risk of infection is low, and if meticulous attention is paid to aseptic techniques, then prophylactic antibiotics may be unwarranted. Need can best be determined by placebo-controlled trials. *Goodman* et al. [52] initiated such a study among patients undergoing both cardiopulmonary bypass and nonbypass procedures. Individuals were randomly assigned to receive placebo, penicillin plus streptomycin, or oxacillin. All 7 life-threatening infections occurred among the 41 patients undergoing cardiopulmonary bypass. 2 patients in the placebo group developed endocarditis, 1 due to *S. pneumoniae* and 1 due to both pneumococcus and penicillin-sensitive staphylococcus. 2 patients developed endocarditis in the penicillin-streptomycin group, and 3 in the oxacillin group. There was no statistically significant reduction in the rate of endocarditis by using antimicrobial prophylaxis. The organisms causing infection were resistant to the antimicrobial prophylaxis employed in 3 of the 4 patients from whom bacteria were isolated. The study was discontinued because the overall results were considered unsatisfactory. This is the only placebo-controlled trial conducted among patients having prosthetic valves implanted. No definite conclusions were reached.

The rationale which has developed for antimicrobial prophylaxis in prosthetic valve surgery may be summarized as follows. Although the risk of infection is low, the consequences of an infection are life-threatening. Safe antibiotics are available which may confer some protection (of particular note were the 2 cases of pneumococcal endocarditis in the placebo group of the study of *Goodman* et al. [52]). Therefore, prophylactic antibiotics should be employed as an adjunctive measure to good surgical technique [53].

In coronary artery bypass graft procedures the scientific evidence for need of antibiotics is more convincing. *Sutherland* et al. [38] reported a postoperative wound infection rate of 0.86% among 693 coronary revascularization procedures without use of systemic antibiotics. However, the mediastinum and pericardium were irrigated with 5% neomycin or 0.4% cephalothin prior to closure. Thus, the authors' statement that operations were performed without antibiotic coverage is not correct. The low incidence of infectious complications is admirable and has not been reproduced by other investigators. But study design limits the relevance of the conclusions. An earlier study by *Sutherland* et al. [54] not only included administration of local antibiotics, but also interjected an additional variable of different surgical teams. Lack of need for antimicrobial prophylaxis was not proven, despite the authors' claims.

Slonim et al. [55] reported a study of 94 patients divided into three groups. The first received placebo (n=16), the next received antibiotics immediately after completion of surgery (n=35), and the third group received antibiotics beginning 12–14 h before surgery. The study suffers from major methodologic problems, not the least of which was non-randomization. But in the recipients of placebo there were 4 staphylococcal bacteremias, 2 wound abscesses and 1 *Pseudomonas* bacteremia. Preoperative administration of antibiotics significantly lessened total infections and staphylococcal infections.

Austin et al. [56] provided some of the best evidence for need of antimicrobial prophylaxis. Patients undergoing coronary artery bypass graft procedures were randomly assigned to receive placebo or cephalothin. The study was terminated after 15 patients because major infectious complications occurred in 4. When the code was broken it was found that all 4 had received placebo, that the infections were caused by staphylococci, and that the phage types of the isolates differed, indicating lack of a common source. Individual patients most likely served as the reservoir for their own wound contamination. The authors concluded that prophylaxis was warranted.

A second placebo-controlled, prospective, double-blind study was conducted by *Fong* et al. [57]. Patients were assigned to receive methicillin or placebo. A total of 132 patients were enrolled, but 27 were excluded for various reasons; 58 received methicillin and 47 received placebo. There were no sternal wound infections in the methicillin group and 10 in the placebo group. 7 of the 10 infections were caused by *S. aureus*. The infections were described as moderate to severe, and there was a significant extension of hospital stay related to this complication. Remote-site infections were also seen in the placebo group. The total number of infections was significantly higher among placebo recipients than in patients receiving methicillin prophylaxis (24 vs. 5; $p < 0.001$).

Additional reports have focused on comparative trials, and assumed that the need for antimicrobial prophylaxis has been established. *Hirschmann and Inui* [53] reviewed prophylaxis trials conducted between 1968 and 1979 for appropriateness of design and validity of conclusions. A study had to be characterized by: (1) prospective data collection; (2) concurrent controls; (3) random allocation of subjects to experimental groups; (4) blind assessment of outcome; (5) precise definitions of outcome and complications; (6) defined criteria for selection of patients; (7) statistical analysis of data, and (8) standardization of the protocol if multiple institutions participated in the study. They identified no study of antimicrobial prophylaxis in open-heart surgery which fulfilled these objectives.

If concurrent controls are taken as patients given an antibiotic considered the 'standard of care' (such as methicillin, cephalothin, or cefazolin) then some studies have adhered to these criteria. The best of the recent trials are summarized in table III. Most authors report no statistical difference in outcome when a new antibiotic is compared with previously available agents alone or in combination.

The study of *Myerowitz* et al. [58] warrants several comments. There were 11 cases of sepsis and/or PVE among recipients of methicillin, none among recipients of cephalothin ($p < 0.001$). There were also significantly more remote-site infections in the methicillin group. The duration of surgery was longer in the cephalothin group, theoretically conferring excess risk of postoperative infection. The conclusion of the study was that cephalothin was a better choice as a prophylactic agent because of its gram-positive and its gram-negative spectrum of activity. The study was not randomized, nor can it be determined whether a blinded evaluation of outcomes was conducted. But the results strongly support the authors' conclusion.

Table III. Comparative trials of antibiotic prophylaxis in open heart surgery

Authors	Reference	Prospective design	Random allocation	Blinded assessment	Defined outcomes	Comparative antibiotics	Statistical difference in outcome
Myerowitz et al.	58	yes	no[1]	not stated	yes	methicillin cephalothin	yes
Kini et al.	99	yes	yes	yes	no	cefazolin cephalothin	no
Pien et al.	100	yes	no[2]	no	yes	clindamycin cephalothin	no
Archer et al.	101	yes	yes	not stated	no	cephalothin cefamandole	no
Cooper et al.	102	yes	no	not stated	not stated	cefazolin penicillin/ flucloxacillin/ streptomycin	no
Bailey and Percival	103	yes	yes[3]	not stated	not stated	penicillin/ flucloxacillin cefamandole	no
Ghonheim et al.	59	yes	yes	not stated	yes	cefamandole ampicillin/ cloxacillin	yes[4]
Parr and Aber	104	yes	yes	yes	yes	cefamandole cephalothin	no
Bryant et al.	105	no	no	no	no	cephalothin cephapirin	no
Raab et al.	43	yes	yes	yes	yes	ceforanide cephalothin	no
Karney et al.	106	yes	yes	yes	yes	cefornide cephalothin	no
Beam et al.	44	yes	yes	yes	yes	ceftriaxone cefazolin	no

[1] Assigned by hospital number.
[2] Alternate assignment to prophylaxis group.
[3] Several protocol violations; planned study not completed.
[4] Method of analysis not given.

The other study reporting a statistical difference in outcomes was conducted by *Ghonheim* et al. [59]. It has several limitations. Patients underwent several different types of surgical procedures. It is not clear how outcomes were assessed. And the total number of patients is small. Statistical significance is only achieved by combining infections of all types and surgical procedures of all types. A clear-cut advantage for cefamandole was not actually proven.

All other studies summarized in table III demonstrated no advantage in terms of reduction of postoperative wound infections for the new antibiotic compared to the old. Our most recent trial involved a comparison of ceftriaxone and cefazolin [44]. Although there was no statistical difference in the rate of infection, there were no infections caused by gram-negative bacilli among patients receiving ceftriaxone. Recipients of cefazolin sustained 1 case of mediastinitis and 1 symptomatic urinary tract infection caused by *Enterobacter* spp. This observation supports the contention of *Myerowitz* et al. [58] that expanded gram-negative activity of the prophylactic agent may confer advantage.

In conclusion, the rationale for antimicrobial prophylaxis in open-heart surgery is based on the studies of *Burke*. Need for antibiotics has not been proven in prosthetic valve surgery. But antibiotics are endorsed and employed in anticipation of a reduced rate of PVE. Evidence is available in coronary artery bypass graft surgery which demonstrates a reduction in postoperative infections when antibiotics are used. Comparative trials of older and newer antibiotics have shown a reduction of gram-negative infections with certain antibiotics. But statistical validation is lacking. Based on the bacteriology of postoperative wound infections, prophylactic antibiotics should be effective against staphylococci and gram-negative bacilli.

Duration of Antimicrobial Prophylaxis

From previously cited work it is apparent that prophylactic antibiotics must be present in concentrations exceeding the MIC of anticipated pathogens during the operative procedure. Numerous recent studies document the distribution characteristics of newer antibiotics and speculate that prophylactic efficacy should occur if the agent were used clinically [60–68]. But demonstrating efficacy was not an objective of these reports.

Of greater interest and potential clinical importance is the observation that the serum half-life of a variety of cephalosporin antibiotics is extended during cardiopulmonary bypass. *Williams and Steele* [69] first made this observation with cephalothin. It was subsequently confirmed for cefamandole [70], cefazolin [71], cephapirin [72], and cefora-nide [73]. The half-life of the drug established in normal volunteers is approximately doubled among patients undergoing cardiopulmonary bypass. Since hemodilution is minimized by current technology, i.e., the pump no longer has to be 'primed' with two units of blood, there is negligible decline in serum concentrations when the patient is placed on bypass. The reason for the prolongation of half-life is unknown.

We found that a cephalosporin such as ceftriaxone, which has a serum half-life of approximately 8 h in normal volunteers [74], has a 16-hour serum half-life among patients on cardiopulmonary bypass [44]. Concentrations of drug in the serum were maintained in excess of the MIC of anticipated pathogens throughout surgery and the early postoperative period after a single 1-gram dose. The drug was delivered by anesthesia personnel in the immediate preoperative period.

Only two studies have been conducted which critically appraise the duration of antibiotic administration necessary for effective prophylaxis in open-heart surgery. *Goldman* et al. [75] compared a 2-day with a 6-day course of cephalothin prophylaxis. Patients received 2-gram doses at 6-hourly intervals. There were 2 sternal wound infections in the short-term prophylaxis group; both were caused by *S. aureus*. There were 3 sternal wound infections in the 6-day prophylaxis group, 2 caused by *S. aureus* and 1 by enterococcus. Remote-site infections were evenly distributed between the two groups. No advantage was demonstrated for continuation of postoperative 'prophylaxis' for 4 additional days.

Conte et al. [76] compared single-dose cephalothin administered intraoperatively with 20 doses administered at 6-hour intervals beginning approximately 12 h preoperatively. 6 of 30 patients having single-dose and 5 of 34 having multiple-dose prophylaxis developed major infectious complications. Pneumonia was the most common process. Only 1 wound infection occurred in each group. Thus, there was no significant difference in infection rates between the two groups. The overall infection rates were relatively high and may be explained by use of 1-gram rather than 2-gram interval doses [61].

The need for long-term antimicrobial prophylaxis in open heart surgery has never been proven. Early studies reported that patients were given antibiotics until discharge from the hospital. More recent efforts have been directed toward short-term prophylaxis. The impact of prophylactic agents on nosocomial flora must always be a cause for concern. Use of a narrow-spectrum antimicrobial is likely to minimize colonization of the individual undergoing surgery by resistant strains [77]. Furthermore, *Archer and Armstrong* [78] have shown that the choice of prophylactic agents may impact the flora of the hospital as a whole.

A balance must therefore be reached. Antimicrobial prophylaxis is widely used in open-heart surgery. It is unlikely that any further placebo-controlled trials will be conducted to document need. There is no proven advantage of long-term antimicrobial use among these patients. But there may be detrimental impact on the individual patient as well as the hospital flora. Short-term prophylaxis, and probably single-dose prophylaxis, is all that is necessary [79]. Antibiotics having a half-life of 2 h or longer need only be administered in a single preoperative dose, even during a lengthy surgical procedure. With drugs having a serum half-life of 1 h or less, a second dose of drug should be given 4 h after the procedure has begun [27].

Reducing Costs of Preventive Therapy in Open Heart Surgery

From the perspective of infection control, as well as economic considerations, new equipment, new devices or new air filtration systems must be proven effective before they are accepted as beneficial to patient care. Simultaneous implementation of several infection control measures has prevented an accurate appraisal of the value of most of the changes in the operating theater now accepted as good standards of care. Cost/benefit ratios cannot be determined.

The area most amenable to cost control is abuse of antimicrobial prophylaxis. *Faden* [80] surveyed 23 pediatric cardiovascular surgery programs for compliance with *Medical Letter* recommendations [81]. Cephalosporins were employed in 74% of procedures. The first dose was given preoperatively 90% of the time. Although no patient received antibiotics longer than 10 days, 51% of patients received antibiotics longer than 3 days. *Medical Letter* guidelines suggest that 72 h should be the maximum duration of antimicrobial prophylaxis. Thus, half of the patients received unnecessary antibiotics.

Crossley and Gardner [82] prospectively evaluated 1021 surgical procedures from 27 hospitals in Minnesota. 62 patients had cardiovascular or thoracic operations. The average duration of prophylaxis was 4.3 days; 52% of patients received antibiotics longer than 3 days. Only 18% had antibiotics given within 4 h preoperatively and terminated within 72 h, that is within the recommended guidelines. Among surgical specialities, the cost per patient for prophylactic antibiotics was highest on cardiothoracic surgery at US$ 82.87/day. The excess expenditure for unwarranted antibiotics was US$ 1,894.02 for the 62 patients evaluated in this study. Since many centers having cardiothoracic surgery perform 100–300 operations per year, the savings which could result from appropriate use of prophylactic antibiotics are substantial.

Fry et al. [83] evaluated compliance with guidelines for antimicrobial prophylaxis at the University of Louisville. Four different procedures were chosen for analysis, including aortofemoral reconstruction. No cardiothoracic procedures were included in their evaluation. But their observation is extremely important. That is, the duration of prophylactic antibiotics was uniformly in violation of the concept of limited postoperative administration.

Kaiser et al. [84] have recently published a cost-benefit analysis for antimicrobial prophylaxis in clean vascular surgery. Cefazolin prophylaxis was given to 225 patients; none developed an infection due to cefazolin-sensitive organisms. 13 patients among 227 recipients of placebo had wound infections. Hospital costs for care were dependent on the severity of infection and ranged from US$ 3,600 to US$ 6,200 per patient. The monetary break-even point was determined to be a rate of 0.5% serious infections, 2.1% moderate infections or 2.4% mild infections. Actual rates of infection exceeded all these values in the placebo group, thus justifying the use of prophylactic antibiotics. Similar calculations could easily be applied to cardiothoracic surgery, but historical controls would have to be used. Allowing for this limitation, cost comparisons between antibiotics could also be made.

Two recommendations are therefore offered for minimizing the cost of antibiotic prophylaxis in open-heart surgery. The first is to use prophylactic antibiotics for an appropriate interval. Coverage is required briefly before, during, and very briefly after completion of the procedure. The second recommendation is to endorse further evaluation of single-dose prophylaxis. Agents with a serum half-life of 2 h or longer are particularly attractive because they should not require readministration, even during prolonged operative procedures. The extended half-life of cephalosporin antibiotics for patients on cardiopulmonary bypass is well documented. Savings in intravenous administration sets, admixture, personnel time and antibiotic costs per se can be realized.

Conclusions

Of the three potential sources of contamination during open-heart surgery, the patient is most often the resource for infecting bacteria. Operating room personnel play a lesser role, and environmental contamination is very infrequently responsible for postoperative infections. Contamination occurs in most procedures [85].

The initial step in the pathogenesis of an infection is bacterial attachment. Organisms capable of colonizing an individual patient may have a selective advantage over random environmental contaminants. That is, given an opportunity to infect an open wound, strains which colonize a hospitalized patient may possess increased pathogenic potential for that individual. Nonspecific clearance mechanisms (opsonins, antibodies and phagocytes) may suffice to eradicate the small numbers of bacteria contaminating the wound. But these measures could be inadequate to deal with carrier strains which possess this attachment quality.

In prosthetic valve surgery, host defenses are compromised by placement of foreign material. Organisms of relatively low pathogenic potential become major problems simply because of the presence of the foreign body. But in coronary artery bypass graft surgery organisms causing postoperative infections are those characteristic of nosocomial flora. In the preantibiotic era, streptococci predominated. In the 1950s and 1960s staphylococci gained prominence. In the recent past gram-negative bacilli have assumed a place of importance in postoperative wound infections among patients undergoing open-heart surgery.

To lessen the risk of postoperative infections, antibiotics have been used as prophylactic agents for cardiothoracic surgical procedures.

There has been no proven value in prosthetic valve surgery. The logic is that administration of safe drugs may lessen the risk of infection. It is worthwhile to give many patients antibiotics in order to prevent just one infection, because the consequences of infection are frequently lethal.

Several studies suggest benefit for using prophylactic antibiotics in coronary artery bypass graft surgery. Trials comparing different prophylactic antibiotic regimes have usually shown no difference in outcome or rates of infectious complications. Advantage may be conferred by using an agent which is active against both staphylococci and gram-negative bacilli.

Cephalosporin antibiotics have a prolonged half-life in patients who undergo surgery requiring cardiopulmonary bypass. Because of this, newer cephalosporin antibiotics having a half-life of 2 h or longer should be evaluated as single-dose prophylactic agents in open-heart surgery. Long-term prophylaxis has never conferred advantage and may increase risk for dissemination of antibiotic-resistant strains in the hospital. Short-term prophylaxis, and particularly single-dose prophylaxis, should have significant economic advantage. Efficacy has not been compromised to date in studies evaluating single-dose prophylaxis.

References

1 Gage, A.A.; Dean, D.C.; Schimert, G.; Minsley, N.: Aspergillus infection after cardiac surgery. Archs Surg. *101:* 384–390 (1970).

2 Soots, G.; Leclerc, H.; Pol, A.; Savage, C.; Fieve, R.: Air-borne contamination hazard in open heart surgery. Efficiency of HEPA air filtration and laminar flow. J. cardiovasc. Surg. *23:* 155–162 (1982).

3 Lidwell, O.M.: Airborne bacteria and surgical infection. Am. J. Med. *70:* 693–697 (1981).

4 Blakemore, W.S.; McGarrity, G.J.; Thurer, R.J.; Wallace, H.W.; MacVaugh, H.; Coriell, L.L.: Infection by air-borne bacteria with cardiopulmonary bypass. Surgery *70:* 830–838 (1971).

5 Lowbury, E.J.L.; Lidwell, O.M.: Multi-hospital trial on the use of ultra-clean air systems. J.R. Soc. Med. *71:* 800–806 (1978).

6 Tsinzo, M.: Infection control in open heart surgery. Infect. Control urol. Care *6:* 22–26 (1981).

7 Maki, D.G.: The prevention and management of device-related infection in infusion therapy. J. Med. *11:* 239–253 (1980).

8 Weinstein, R.; Emori, T.G.; Anderson, R.L.; Stamm, W.E.: Pressure transducers as a source of bacteremia after heart surgery. Chest *69:* 338–344 (1976).

9 Sanford, J.P.; Pierce, A.K.: Lower respiratory tract infections; in Bennett, Brachman, Hospital infections, pp. 255–286 (Little Brown, Boston 1979).
10 Geldof, W.CH.P.; Brom, A.G.: Infections through blood from heart-lung machine. Thorax *27:* 395–397 (1972).
11 Freeman, R.; Hjersing, N.: Bacterial culture of perfusion blood after open heart surgery. Thorax *35:* 754–758 (1980).
12 Maki, G.G.; Rhame, F.S.; Mackel, D.C.; Bennett, J.V.: Nationwide epidemic of septicemia caused by contaminated intravenous products. I. Epidemiologic and clinical features. Am. J. Med. *60:* 471–485 (1976).
13 Unsigned: Follow-up on nosocomial *Pseudomonas cepacia* infection. Morb. Mortal. Wkly Rep. *28:* 409 (1979).
14 Altman, G.; Horowitz, A.; Kaplinsky, N.; Frankl, O.: Prosthetic valve endocarditis due to *Mycobacterium chelonei*. J. clin. Microbiol. *1:* 531–533 (1975).
15 Robicsek, F.; Daugherty, H.K.; Cook, J.W.; Selle, J.G.; Masters, T.N.; O'Bar, P.R.; Fernandez, C.R.; Mauney, C.U.; Calhoun, D.M.: *Mycobacterium fortuitum* epidemics after open heart surgery. J. thorac. cardiovasc. Surg. *75:* 91–96 (1978).
16 Hughes, R.K.: A method of improved antisepsis for open-heart surgery. Ann. thorac. Surg. *2:* 230–236 (1966).
17 Clark, R.E.; Amos, W.C.; Higgins, V.; Bemberg, P.E.; Weldon, C.S.: Infection control in cardiac surgery. Surgery *79:* 89–96 (1976).
18 Norden, C.W.; Ruben, F.L.: Staphylococcal infections; in Wherle, Top. communicable and infectious diseases, pp. 589–605 (Mosby, St. Louis 1981).
19 Bernard, H.R.; Cole, W.R.: The epidemiology of postoperative surgical infection. Surg. Clins. N. Am. *45:* 509–519 (1965).
20 Burke, J.F.: Identification of the sources of staphylococci contaminating the surgical wound during operation. Ann. Surg. *158:* 898–904 (1963).
21 Howe, C.W.; Marston, A.T.: A study on sources of postoperative staphylococcal infection. Surgery Gynec. Obstet. *115:* 266–275 (1962).
22 Meleney, F.L.: Infection in clean operative wounds. A nine-year study. Surgery Gynec. Obstet. *60:* 264–276 (1935).
23 Beam, T.R.; Bhayana, J.N.; Raab, T.A.; Balderman, S.C.; McDermott, C.A.; Mylotte, J.M.: Failure of antimicrobial prophylaxis in open heart surgery. Clin. Res. *29:* 726A (1981).
24 Simchen, E.; Shapiro, M.; Marin, G.; Sacks, T.; Michel, J.: Risk factors for postoperative wound infection in cardiac surgery patients. Infect. Control *4:* 215–220 (1983).
25 Brown, A.H.; Braimbridge, M.V.; Panagopoulos, P.; Sabar, E.F.: The complications of median sternotomy. J. thorac. cardiovasc. Surg. *58:* 189–197 (1969).
26 Roy, A.C.; Penhall, J.R.H.; Cameron, E.W.J.: Management of disrupted sternotomy. Thorax *36:* 676–678 (1981).
27 Ehrenkranz, N.J.: Surgical wound infection occurrence in clean operations. Risk stratification for interhospital comparisons. Am. J. Med. *70:* 909–914 (1981).
28 Todd, J.C.: Wound infection: etiology, prevention and management. Surg. Clins. N.Am. *48:* 787–798 (1968).
29 Altemeir, W.A.: Surgical infections: incisional wounds; in Bennett, Brachman, Hospital infections, pp. 287–306 (Little Brown, Boston, 1979).

30 Eickoff, T.C.: Antibiotics and nosocomial infections; in Bennett, Brachman, Hospital infections, pp. 195–221 (Little Brown, Boston 1979).
31 Delgado, D.G.; Cobbs, C.G.: Infections of prosthetic valves and intravascular devices; in Mandell, Douglas, Bennett, Principles and practice of infectious diseases, pp. 690–697 (Wiley, New York 1979).
32 Christensen, G.D.; Simpson, W.A.; Bisno, A.L.; Beachey, E.H.: Experimental foreign body infections in mice challenged with slime-producing *Staphylococcus epidermidis*. Infect. Immunity *40:* 407–410 (1983).
33 Peters, G.; Locci, R.; Pulverer, G.: Adherence and growth of coagulase-negative staphylococci on surfaces of intravenous catheters. J. infect. Dis. *146:* 479–482 (1983).
34 Karchmer, A.W.; Archer, G.L.; Dismukes, W.E.: *Staphylococcus epidermidis* causing prosthetic valve endocarditis: microbiologic and clinical observations as guides to therapy. Ann. intern. Med. *98:* 447–455 (1983).
35 Wenzel, R.P.: The emergence of methicillin-resistant *Staphylococcus aureus*. Ann. intern. Med. *97:* 440–442 (1982).
36 DeLaria, G.A.; Hunter, J.A.; Goldin, M.D.; Serry, C.; Javid, H.; Najafi, H.: Leg wound complications associated with coronary revascularization. J. thorac. cardiovasc. Surg. *81:* 403–407 (1981).
37 Bain, W.H.; McGeachie, J.; Lindsay, G.; Underwood, J.: The use of cephalothin sodium (keflin) as the prophylactic antibiotic for open heart surgery. J. antimicrob. Chemother. *3:* 339–345 (1977).
38 Sutherland, R.D.; Martinez, H.E.; Fyfe, T.; Harkrider, W.: Coronary arterial bypass operations without antibiotic coverage. Chest *76:* 174–175 (1979).
39 Wells, F.C.; Newsom, S.W.B.; Rowlands, C.: Wound infection in cardiothoracic surgery. Lancet *i:* 1209–1210 (1983).
40 Farrington, M.; Webster, M.; Fenn, A.; Phillips, I.: Wound infection in cardiothoracic surgery. Lancet *ii:* 395–396 (1983).
41 Johanson, W.G.; Pierce, A.K.; Sanford, J.P.; Thomas, G.D.; Nosocomial respiratory infections with gram-negative bacilli: The significance of colonization of the respiratory tract. Ann. intern. Med. *77:* 701–706 (1972).
42 Johanson, W.G.; Pierce, A.K.; Sanford, J.P.: Changing pharyngeal bacterial flora of hospitalized patients. New Engl. J. Med. *281:* 1137–1140 (1969).
43 Raab, T.A.; Balderman, S.; Bhayana, J.; Bingham, K.; Mylotte, J.; Beam, T.R., Jr.: A comparison of the safety, efficacy and distribution of ceforanide and cephalothin in coronary artery bypass graft surgery. Ann. thorac. Surg. *33:* 340–344 (1982).
44 Beam, T.R.; Raab, T.A.; Spooner, J.A.; Balderman, S.C.; Aldridge, J.; Bhayana, J.N.: Comparison of ceftriaxone and cefazolin prophylaxis against infection in open heart surgery. Am. J. Surg. (in press).
45 O'Brien, T.F.; Ross, D.G.; Gusman, M.A.; Madeiros, A.A.; Hedges, R.W.; Botstein, D.: Dissemination of an antibiotic resistance plasmid in hospital flora. Antimicrob. Agents Chemother. *17:* 537–543 (1980).
46 O'Brien, T.F.; Hopkins, J.D.; Gilleece, E.S.; Madeiros, A.A.; Kent, R.L.; Blackburn, B.O.; Holmes, M.B.; Reardon, J.P.; Vergeront, J.M.; Schell, W.J.; Christenson, T.; Bissett, M.L.; Morse, E.V.: Molecular epidemiology of antibiotic resistance in *Salmonella* from animals and human beings in the United States. New Engl. J. Med. *307:* 1–6 (1982).

47 Williams, E.W.; Hawkey, P.M.; Penner, J.L.; Senior, B.W.; Barton, L.J.: Serious nosocomial infection caused by *Morganella morgagnii* and *Proteus mirabilis* in a cardiac surgery unit. J. clin. Microbiol. *18:* 5–9 (1983).
48 Miles, A.A.; Miles, E.M.; Burke, J.: The value and duration of defence reactions of the skin to the primary lodgement of bacteria. Br. J. exp. Path. *38:* 79–96 (1957).
49 Burke, J.F.: The effective period of preventive antibiotic action in experimental incisions and dermal lesions. Surgery *50:* 161–168 (1961).
50 Dineen, P.: A period of unusual microbial susceptibility in an experimental staphylococcal infection. J. infect. Dis. *108:* 174–180 (1961).
51 Dineen, P.: Further studies on the period of microbial susceptibility. J. infect. Dis. *111:* 169–174 (1962).
52 Goodman, J.S.; Schaffner, W.; Collins, H.A.; Battersby, E.J.; Koenig, M.G.: Infection after cardiovascular surgery. Clinical study including examination of antimicrobial prophylaxis. New Engl. J. Med. *278:* 117–123 (1968).
53 Hirschmann, J.V.; Inui, T.S.: Antimicrobial prophylaxis: a critique of recent trials. Rev. infect. Dis. *2:* 1–23 (1980).
54 Sutherland, R.D.; Martinez, H.E.; Cuynes, W.A.; Miller, L.: Postoperative chest wound infections in patients requiring coronary bypass. A controlled study evaluating prophylactic antibiotics. J. thorac. cardiovasc. Surg. *73:* 944–947 (1977).
55 Slonim, R.; Litwak, R.S.; Gadboys, H.L.; Ehrenkranz, N.J.: Antibiotic prophylaxis of infection complicating open-heart operations. Antimicrob. Agents Chemother. *3:* 731–735 (1963).
56 Austin, T.W.; Coles, J.C.; Burnett, R.; Goldbach, M.: Aortocoronary bypass procedures and sternotomy infections: a study of antistaphylococcal prophylaxis. Can. J. Surg. *23:* 483–485 (1980).
57 Fong, I.W.; Baker, C.B.; McKee, D.C.: The value of prophylactic antibiotics in aorta-coronary bypass operations. A double-blind randomized trial. J. thorac. cardiovasc. Surg. *78:* 908–913 (1979).
58 Myerowitz, P.D.; Caswell, K.; Lindsay, W.G.; Nicoloff, D.M.: Antibiotic prophylaxis for open-heart surgery. J. thorac. cardiovasc. Surg. *73:* 625–629 (1977).
59 Ghonheim, A.T.M.; Tandon, A.P.; Ionescu, M.I.: Comparative study of cefamandole versus ampicillin plus cloxacillin: prophylactic antibiotics in cardiac surgery. Ann. thorac. Surg. *33:* 152–158 (1982).
60 Kluge, R.M.; Calia, F.M.; McLaughlin, J.S.; Hornick, R.B.: Serum antibiotic concentrations pre-and postcardiopulmonary bypass. Antimicrob. Agents Chemother. *4:* 270–276 (1973).
61 Austin, T.W.; Coles, J.C.; McKechnie, P.; Sandoval, W.; Doctor, A.: Cephalothin prophylaxis and valve replacement. Ann. thorac. Surg. *23:* 333–336 (1977).
62 Eigel, P.; Tschirkov, A.; Satter, P.; Knothe, H.: Assays of cephalosporin antibiotics administered prophylactically in open heart surgery. Determination of serum and tissue levels before, during and after cardiopulmonary bypass. Infection *6:* 23–28 (1978).
63 Quintiliani, R.; Klimek, J.; Nightingale, C.H.: Penetration of cephapirin and cephalothin into the right atrial appendage and pericardial fluid of patients undergoing open heart surgery. J. infect. Dis. *139:* 348–352 (1979).
64 Nightingale, C.H.; Klimek, J.J.; Quintiliani, R.: Effect of protein binding on the

penetration of nonmetabolized cephalosporins into atrial appendage and pericardial fluids in open-heart surgical patients. Antimicrob. Agents Chemother. *17:* 595–598 (1980).
65 Daschner, F.D.; Metz, B.; Spillner, G.; Buzello, W.; Schlosser, V.: Concentrations of cefamandole and cefsulodin in serum, heart valves, subcutaneous tissue and muscle of patients undergoing open-heart surgery. *142:* 290 (1980).
66 Daschner, F.D.; Eschenbruch, E.; Metz, B.; Bayer, E.; Schmuziger, M.: Penetration of gentamicin into heart valves subcutaneous and muscular tissue of patients undergoing open heart surgery. J. cardiovasc. Surg. *22:* 581–584 (1981).
67 Daschner, F.D.; Just, M.; Spillner, G.; Schlosser, V.: Penetration of piperacillin into cardiac valves, subcutaneous and muscle tissue of patients undergoing open-heart surgery. J. antimicrob. Chemother. *9:* 489–492 (1982).
68 Sterling, R.P.; Connor, D.J.; Norman, J.C.; Cooley, D.A.: Cefonicid concentrations in serum and atrial tissue during open-heart surgery. Antimicrob. Agents Chemother. *23:* 790–792 (1983).
69 Williams, D.J.; Steele, T.W.: Cephalothin prophylaxis assay during cardiopulmonary bypass. J. thorac. cardiovasc. Surg. *71:* 207–211 (1976).
70 Polk, R.E.; Archer, G.L.; Lower, R.: Cefamandole kinetics during cardiopulmonary bypass. Clin. Pharmacol. Ther. *23:* 473–480 (1978).
71 Miller, K.W.; McCoy, H.G.; Chan, K.K.H.; Fischer, R.P.; Lindsay, W.G.; Seifert, R.D.; Zaske, D.E.: Effect of cardiopulmonary bypass on cefazolin disposition. Clin. Pharmacol. Ther. *27:* 550–556 (1980).
72 Green, E.R.; Subramanian, S.; Faden, H.; Quintiliani, R.; Nightingale, C.H.: A comparison of the penetration characteristics of cephapirin and cephalothin into right atrial appendage, muscle, fat, and pericardial fluid of pediatric patients undergoing open-heart operation. Ann. thorac. Surg. *31:* 155–160 (1981).
73 Mullany, L.D.; French, M.A.; Nightingale, C.H.; Low, H.B.C.; Ellison, L.H.; Quintiliani, R.: Penetration of ceforanide and cefamandole into the right atrial appendage, pericardial fluid, sternum and intercostal muscle of patients undergoing open heart surgery. Antimicrob. Agents Chemother. *21:* 416–420 (1982).
74 Patel, I.H.; Chen, S.; Parsonnet, M.; Hackman, M.R.; Brooks, M.A.; Konikoff, J.; Kaplan, S.A.: Pharmacokinetics of ceftriaxone in humans. Antimicrob. Agents Chemother. *20:* 634–641 (1981).
75 Goldman, D.A.; Hopkins, C.C.; Karchmer, A.W.; Abel, R.M.; McEnany, T.; Akins, C.; Buckley, M.J.; Moellering, R.C.: Cephalothin prophylaxis in cardiac valve surgery. A prospective, double-blind comparison of two-day and six-day regimens. J. thorac. cardiovasc, Surg. *73:* 470–479 (1977).
76 Conte, J.E.; Cohen, S.N.; Roe, B.B.; Elashoff, R.M.: Antibiotic prophylaxis and cardiac surgery. A prospective double-blind comparison of single-dose versus multiple-dose regimens. Ann. intern. Med. *76:* 943–949 (1972).
77 Freeman, R.: Short-term adverse effects of antibiotic prophylaxis for open heart surgery. Thorax *35:* 941–944 (1980).
78 Archer, G.L.; Armstrong, B.C.: Alteration of staphylococcal flora in cardiac surgery patients receiving antibiotic prophylaxis. J. infect. Dis. *147:* 642–649 (1983).
79 Beam, T.R.; Raab, T.A.; Spooner, J.A.; Balderman, S.C.; Aldridge, J.; Bhayana, J.N.: Single dose antimicrobial prophylaxis in open heart surgery. Eur. J. clin. Microbiol. (in press).

80 Faden, H.: Prophylactic antibiotics in pediatric cardiovascular surgery: current practices. Ann. thorac. surg. *31:* 211–213 (1981).
81 Unsigned: Antimicrobial prophylaxis for surgery. Med. Lett. *23:* 77–80 (1981).
82 Crossley, K.; Gardner, L.C.: Antimicrobial prophylaxis in surgical patients. J. Am. med. Ass. *245:* 722–726 (1981).
83 Fry, D.E.; Harbrecht, P.J.; Polk, H.C.: Systemic prophylactic antibiotics. Need the 'cost' be so high? Archs Surg. *116:* 466–469 (1981).
84 Kaiser, A.B.; Roach, A.C.; Mulherin, J.L.; Clayson, K.R.; Allen, T.R.; Edwards, W.H.; Dale, W.A.: The cost effectiveness of antimicrobial prophylaxis in clean vascular surgery. J. infect. Dis. *147:* 1103–1107 (1983).
85 Kluge, R.M.; Calia, F.M.; McLaughlin, J.S.; Hornick, R.B.: Sources of contamination in open heart surgery. J. Am. med. Ass. *230:* 1415–1418 (1974).
86 Amoury, R.A.; Bowman, F.A., Jr.; Malm, J.R.: Endocarditis associated with intracardiac prosthesis. J. thorac. cardiovasc. Surg. *51:* 36–48 (1966).
87 Stein, P.D.; Harken, D.E.; Dester, L.: The nature and prevention of prosthetic valve endocarditis. Am. Heart J. *71:* 393–407 (1966).
88 Dismukes, W.E.; Karchmer, A.W.; Buckley, M.J.; Austin, W.G.; Swartz, M.N.: Prostehtic valve endocarditis. Circulation *48:* 365–377 (1973).
89 Slaughter, L.; Morris, J.E.; Starr, A.: Prosthetic valve endocarditis. Circulation *47:* 1319–1326 (1973).
90 Wilson, W.R.; Jaumin, P.M.; Danielson, G.K.; Giuliani, E.R.; Washington, J.A. II; Geraci, J.E.: Prosthetic valve endocarditis. Ann. intern. Med. *82:* 751–756 (1975).
91 Aintablian, A.; Hilsemath, J.; Hamby, R.I.; Sancet, C.M.; Hartstein, M.L.; Wisoff, B.G.: Endocarditis in prosthetic valves. N. Y. St. J. Med. *76:* 673–677 (1976).
92 Rossiter, S.J.; Stinson, E.B.; Dyer, P.E.; Miller, D.C.; Schapira, J.W.; Martin, R.P.; Shumway, N.E.: Prosthetic valve endocarditis: comparison of heterograft tissue valves and mechanical valves. J. thorac. cardiovasc. Surg. *76:* 795–802 (1978).
93 Masur, H.; Johnson, W.D., Jr.: Prosthetic valve endocarditis. J. thorac. cardiovasc. Surg. *80:* 31–37 (1980).
94 Sanfelippo, P.M.; Danielson, G.K.: Complications associated with median sternotomy. J. thorac. cardiovasc. Surg. *63:* 419–423 (1972).
95 Engelman, R.M.; Williams, C.D.; Gouge, T.H.; Chase, R.M., Jr.; Falk, E.A.; Boyd, A.D.; Reed, G.E.: Mediastinitis following open-heart surgery. Review of two years' experience. Archs Surg. *107:* 772–778 (1973).
96 Culliford, A.T.; Cunningham, J.N., Jr.; Zeff, R.H.; Isom, O.W.; Teiko, P.; Spencer, F.C.: Sternal and costochondral infections following open heart surgery. A review of 2,594 cases. J. thorac. cardiovasc. Surg. *72:* 714–726 (1976).
97 Stoney, W.S.; Alford, W.C., Jr.; Burrus, G.R.; First, R.A.; Thomas, C.S., Jr.: Median sternotomy dehiscence. Ann. thorac. Surg. *26:* 421–426 (1978).
98 Bor, D.H.; Rose, R.M.; Modlin, J.F.; Weintraub, R.; Friedland, G.H.: Mediastinitis after cardiovascular surgery. Rev. infect. Dis. *5:* 885–897 (1983).
99 Kini, P.M.; Fernandez, J.; Causay, R.S.; Lemole, G.M.: Double-blind comparison of cefazolin and cephalothin in open heart surgery. J. thorac. cardiovasc. Surg. *76:* 506–509 (1978).
100 Pien, F.D.; Michael, N.L.; Mamiya, R.; Takaki, H.; Slavish, S.; Bruce, A.; Moreno-Cabral, R.J.: Comparative study of prophylactic antibiotics in cardiac surgery. Clindamycin versus cephalothin. J. thorac. cardiovasc. Surg. *77:* 908–913 (1979).

101 Archer, G.L.; Polk, R.E.; Duma, R.J.; Lower, R.: Comparison of cephalothin and cefamandole prophylaxis during insertion of prosthetic heart valves. Antimicrob. Agents Chemother. *13:* 924–929 (1978).
102 Cooper, D.K.C.; Norton, R.; Mobin, M.A.; Cleland, W.P.; Bentall, H.H.; Darrell, J.H.: A comparison of two prophylactic antibiotic regimes for open-heart surgery. J. cardiovasc. Surg. *21:* 279–286 (1980).
103 Bailey, J.S.; Percival, H.G.: Cefamandole as a prophylactic in cardiac surgery. Scand. J. infect. Dis. *S25:* 112–117 (1980).
104 Parr, G.V.S.; Aber, R.C.: Comparative efficacy and tolerance of cefamandole and cephalothin as prophylaxis for open heart surgery: a randomized double-blind study. J. cardiovasc. Surg. *23:* 305–308 (1982).
105 Bryant, R.E.; Hartstein, A.I.; Starr, A.; Beals, R.K.: Chemoprophylaxis in cardiac orthopedic surgery: Comparison of cephalothin and cephapirin. Sth. med. J. *75:* 1057–1062 (1982).
106 Karney, W.; Correa-Coronas, R.; Zajtchuk, R.; Schwartz, J.; Smith, L.P.; Tramont, E.: Comparion of cephalothin and ceforanide prophylaxis in cardiac surgery with cardiopulmonary bypass. Antimicrob. Agents Chemother. *24:* 85–88 (1983).

T.R. Beam, Jr., MD, Chief, Infectious Diseases (111F), VA Medical Center,
3495 Bailey Avenue, Buffalo, NY 14215 (USA)

Antibiot. Chemother., vol. 33, pp. 140–164 (Karger, Basel 1985)

Prevention of Infection Following Orthopedic Surgery

Lawrence J. Eron

Division of Infectious Diseases, The Fairfax Hospital, Falls Church, Va., USA

Infection following orthopedic surgery can be a devastating event. It may result in a lifelong non-union of a fracture, a totally unusable joint, chronic pain or amputation. In order to minimize the chance of infection following certain orthopedic procedures, antibiotics are commonly used perioperatively. To determine the most effective manner in which antibiotics may be used in the prevention of infection, it is worthwhile to consider how infection may occur in orthopedic settings.

The development of an infection following orthopedic surgery depends on either the direct inoculation of bacteria into wounds or the seeding of bones or joints via hematogenous dissemination. The bacterial inoculum at first colonizes the bone, joint, or wound without inflammation. *Colonization* may develop into a bona fide *infection* depending on the size of the bacterial inoculum, the status of the host, and the type of bacteria inoculated into the wound.

Inoculum Size

A wound, whether hematogenously seeded, or traumatically or surgically induced, may be categorized according to the size of the bacterial inoculum. Clean wounds have a small inoculum of bacteria as would occur in most elective orthopedic surgery. Contaminated wounds range from clean-contaminated with a moderate inoculum to frankly dirty with a heavy inoculum, as would occur in a motorcycle accident in which debris is driven directly into the wound. The goal of prophylaxis is to reduce the inoculum of contaminating bacteria, for the larger the inoculum, the greater the likelihood that colonization of the wound will lead to infection. With appropriate care even the dirtiest wounds can be cleansed of the colonizing bacteria to prevent subsequent infection.

Host Factors

The most important host factor determining whether bacterial contamination of a wound will produce an infection is the condition of the tissues, which can range from healthy to ischemic or frankly necrotic. The less viable the tissue is, the more likely bacteria will invade it. The presence of hematoma formation within a wound is also a favorable environment for bacterial growth. Foreign bodies may allow ordinarily nonpathogenic bacteria such as *Staphylococcus epidermidis* to cause infection. In addition to the tissues within the wound, the host's age, nutritional status, and the presence of underlying disease such as diabetes mellitus, sickle cell anemia, rheumatoid arthritis, uremia, cirrhosis, or steroid therapy may further complicate things. These diseases may affect the body's ability to mobilize polymorphonuclear leukocytes to the wounds, to ingest the bacteria, and to kill the bacteria. Specific hereditary and acquired deficiencies of immunoglobulin and complement may also interfere with the host's ability to control contamination of a wound.

Bacteriology

The choice of a prophylactic antibiotic must be based on the types of bacteria likely to cause a wound infection. Those infections that occur following elective orthopedic surgery principally involve *Staphylococcus aureus, S. epidermidis,* and *Streptococcus* spp. Other bacteria besides these may cause infection. Wounds of the lower extremities may become infected by gram-negative bacilli. Puncture wounds of the foot are frequently inoculated with *Pseudomonas aeruginosa.* Gram-negative bacillary infection may also occur in patients with open wounds initially infected with *S. aureus, S. epidermidis,* or *Streptococcus* spp. The infection may be treated appropriately with a semisynthetic penicillin or cephalosporin, but then resistant organisms such as *Serratia, Enterobacter*, or *Pseudomonas* may secondarily invade the wound. Lacerations sustained in rivers have a special inclination to become infected with *Aeromonas hydrophila.* Animal bites are often infected with *Pasteurella multocida*, a penicillin-sensitive but cephalothin-resistant organism. When tissues become ischemic, anaerobic organisms may predominate. Patients with diabetes mellitus may develop pedal ulcers infected by polymicrobial flora including anaerobic and facultative gram-negative bacilli.

A rational choice of an antibiotic for prophylaxis must be made on the basis of the knowledge of the bacteriology of each particular situation. However, when one is not sure what the offending organism is in a potentially contaminated wound, it is wise to culture the wound and to obtain a gram-stained specimen. If one notes a homogeneous type of organism amongst polymorphonuclear leukocytes, one can act immediately on that information without awaiting the culture results [13].

In determining the probability of infection, it has been estimated using animal models that 10^5 colonies of *S. aureus* is the critical level necessary to establish a wound infection [63]. In human volunteers, higher titers of 7×10^6 colonies are required to produce infection [20]. Yet most authors agree that the average inoculum into wounds during elective orthopedic surgical procedures occurs at the rate of only about 10^2 colonies/h [5, 36, 48, 76]. How do we explain such a discrepancy between these figures? Animal data suggest that ischemia will allow several thousand times fewer bacteria to produce a wound infection [45]. Indeed, in humans, a dose of 7.5×10^6 colonies of *S. aureus* is required to produce infection by intradermal injection in human volunteers but only 3×10^3 organisms are required if a foreign body such as a silk stitch is inserted as well [21].

Sources of Infection

Infection can result from the inoculation of bacteria into a wound (from an exogenous source) or from hematogenous dissemination (from an endogenous source within the body). Exogenous sources of contamination generally include bacteria from the patient's skin, bacteria on weapons or on surgical instruments, or fallout from the air. Endogenous sources of bacteria may contaminate wounds by hematogenous spread from a separate site of infection in the patient such as a skin or soft-tissue infection which may be as trivial as a boil, a dental infection, a urinary tract infection, or a respiratory tract infection. Generally, with adequate preoperative screening, early infection due to endogenous sources can be avoided. However, late infections may seed prostheses up to several years after their insertion [7, 45, 70, 75]. Patients should be made aware of this fact and infection elsewhere in their body should be promptly diagnosed and treated. For all practical purposes, exogenous sources are the principal ones of concern.

In the preparation of wounds for surgery, it should be understood that wounds are always contaminated to a greater or lesser degree at the time of the incision. Although bacteria may be removed fairly easily from the epidermis, they cannot be sterilized from hair follicles or sebaceous glands in which they normally reside. Skin disinfectants penetrate poorly into these areas, which can never be totally disinfected. However, the number of bacteria can be reduced by careful attention to the preparation of the operative site. On the day prior to surgery, only washing of the operative area is performed. Iodophors are utilized preoperatively and shaving is performed, only when necessary, immediately preoperatively. Correct draping, separating the operative area from potentially dirty areas such as the genitals and the anus, and correct gowning and double gloving are also important. Impervious disposable fabric is used for drapes and gowns where possible.

Contamination from the Air

In conventional operating rooms, air intake may be filtered only minimally and with only 10 to 25 exchanges of air per hour, particles may settle onto the operating field or instruments. Newer operating rooms, utilizing laminar airflow with as many as 300 changes of air per hour through a series of filters of progressively smaller pores to screen out particulate matter, reduce the number of particles in the air from more than 50 per m^3 of air to less than 5. This may in turn reduce the bacterial inoculum into the wounds as well.

Various investigators [9, 11, 41] were able to reduce infection rates from 7–10% to less than 1% for joint replacements, utilizing ultraclean airflow through high-efficiency particulate air filters. Other factors that are important for air quality include a decrease in the amount of traffic into and out of the operating room as well as minimizing circulating personnel within the operating room. By these measures, lower bacterial counts can be obtained on plates that are left open to the air to allow bacteria to settle on them.

In an attempt to decrease the number of viable bacteria, ultraviolet light has been utilized to produce ultraclean air. However, there is some controversy as to its utility [29]. The use of total-body exhaust systems has also been advocated [41] but the cost effectiveness of this suggestion is not yet clear.

While air quality is undoubtedly important, there must be other important considerations in addition to fall-out of bacteria from the air into the wound. Infection rate does not always correlate with the results of these surveillance plates [34], and the settling of bacteria into the wound does not mean that an infection will be established. In one series of hip replacements [12], a piece of tissue from the hip capsule was cultured routinely and found to be positive in 25% of cases, even though there was not one case of deep infection in this series. *Salvatti* et al. [68] failed to note any benefit from the use of ultraclean air in total joint replacements, and *Coventry* et al. [15] found a 0.6% infection rate in total hip arthroplasties inserted without laminar airflow.

Timing and Duration of Prophylaxis

It has been amply shown that in order to obtain the maximal prophylactic effect, the antibiotic must be given in time to have adequate tissue levels at the moment of wound contamination. The prophylactic effect of the antibiotic may be lost if it is administered 4 h or longer after the incision is made [5].

When bacteria colonize a wound, polymorphonuclear leukocytes and macrophages are mobilized to the site of contamination to remove the bacteria. After a period of 4–6 h of little or no growth (the stationary period), if contamination is not too extensive, the bacteria begin multiplying at a rate less than that by which they are killed by the host defense mechanisms. If the wound is grossly contaminated, there may be too many bacteria such that they begin multiplying faster than they can be removed. In this case, if antibiotics are added at the end of the first 6 h following contamination, the bacteria may be growing too rapidly to be controlled. Yet, if grossly contaminated wounds are irrigated free of debris, antibiotics added during the first several hours of contamination may assist the host defense mechanisms in overwhelming heavy bacterial contamination.

A brief period of antibiotic prophylaxis is desirable from the standpoints of cost, side effects, and overgrowth of resistant flora. The longer an antibiotic is used, the greater the opportunity for resistant flora to colonize the wounds. In early studies by *Ericson* et al. [22] and *Carlsson* et al. [8], cloxacillin was prophylactically administered postoperatively for 2 weeks in patients undergoing total hip replacements. Subsequent studies by *Schulitz* et al. [69] reduced the duration to 10 days for lincomycin and to 5 days in a study by *Hill* et al. [34] utilizing cefazolin. Finally, *Pollard* et al. [61] showed that the prophylactic efficacy of merely three doses of cephaloridine was as effective as 14 days of flucloxacillin. These results were confirmed by *Nelson* et al. [49] who compared 7 days to 1 of nafcillin or cefazolin in total joint replacement and hip fracture repair. Future studies may show that a single dose of antibiotic prevents infection in total hip replacement.

Choice of Antibiotics

The prophylactic antibiotic chosen must be active against the particular bacteria targeted and should possess as narrow an antibacterial spectrum as possible. It should be able to penetrate into hematoma, joint, and bone where bacterial contamination has occurred or will occur. A prophylactic antibiotic should have a small likelihood of causing an adverse drug reaction, and should be relatively inexpensive.

The antibiotics used in orthopedic surgery for prophylaxis include the semisynthetic penicillins such as nafcillin, oxacillin, cloxacillin, and flucloxacillin, as well as the 'first-generation' cephalosporins including cephalothin, cefazolin, cephradine, and cephapirin (table I). These groups of antibiotics have a number of things in common, the most important of which is their activity against *S. aureus, S. epidermidis,* and *Streptococcus* spp., the prime pathogens in infections involving prostheses. The new cephalosporins (table II), the so-called 'second-generation' (cefoxitin and cefamandole) and 'third-generation' (moxalactam, cefoperazone, and cefotaxime) cephalosporins, are not useful for orthopedic prophylaxis unless resistant gram-negative bacilli are expected.

Table I. Antibiotics useful in prophylaxis

	Dosage[a]	Spectrum of activity	Daily cost[b] US $	Toxicity
Cefazolin	1 g/6 h[c]	excellent for *S. aureus, S. epidermidis, Strep., E. coli, Klebsiella*	13.20	rash, rare leukopenia
Nafcillin	1 g/4 h	excellent for *S. aureus* and *Strep.;* only fair for *S. epidermidis*	8.40	rash, rare leukopenia
Vancomycin	0.5 g/6 h[c]	excellent for *S. aureus, S. epidermidis* and *Strep.*	70.28	renal and ototoxicity
Clindamycin	0.6 g/6 h	excellent for *S. aureus, Strep.* and anaerobes; only fair for *S. epidermidis*	44.36	rash, rare enterocolitis
Gentamicin	1.5 mg/ kg/ 8 h[c]	excellent for virtually all gram-negative bacilli; fair for *S. aureus;* poor for *Strep.*	2.92	renal and ototoxicity

[a] Suggested dosages from the respective pharmaceutical companies.
[b] Acquisition costs of the Fairfax Hospital.
[c] For reduced creatinine clearance, the frequency of administration should be reduced.

In patients who are allergic to cephalosporins, the use of vancomycin has been advocated, although this drug is expensive and may be ototoxic and nephrotoxic. Other possible alternatives include clindamycin which has good activity against *S. aureus* but only fair activity against *S. epidermidis.* Penicillin, ampicillin, ticarcillin, mezlocillin, and piperacillin (table II) have not been utilized because of high-grade resistance by most *Staphylococcus* spp. Erythromycin, while active against the majority of *S. aureus* infections, has been little utilized in prophylactic situations, as it is not well tolerated intravenously, causing phlebitis.

Recently, *S. epidermidis* [42] and to a lesser degree *S. aureus* [79] have become increasingly resistant to the semisynthetic penicillins

Table II. Third-generation β-lactam antibiotics

	Dosage[a]	Spectrum of activity	Daily cost[b] US $	Gaps in spectrum
Cefotaxime[c]	2 g/6 h	*S. aureus, Strep.*, most gram-negative bacilli	75.44	fair to poor for *P. aeruginosa, S. fecalis, Enterobacter, S. epidermidis*
Ceftriaxone	1 g/24 h		NA	
Cefoperazone	2 g/12 h		37.32	
Moxalactam	2 g/12 h		52.80	
Cefsulodin	1 g/6 h	*S. aureus* and *P. aeruginosa*	NA	*Strep.*, anaerobes, all other gram-negative bacilli, *S. fecalis*
Ceftazidime	1 g/8 h	*Serratia, P. aeruginosa*, and most gram-negative bacilli	NA	only fair for *Enterobacter* and *S. aureus*, poor for *S. epidermidis, S. fecalis*
Imipenem	0.5 g/6 h	*S. aureus, S. epidermidis, Strep.* (including *S. fecalis*), anaerobes, and most gram-negative bacilli	NA	only fair for *Enterobacter*
Azlocillin	3 g/4 h	*Strep.* (including *S. fecalis*), *P. aeruginosa*, and most gram-negative bacilli	73.80	*S. aureus, S. epidermidis*
Piperacillin	3 g/4 h		63.36	
Mezlocillin	3 g/4 h		55.84	

[a] Therapeutic dosages suggested by the respective pharmaceutical companies.
[b] Acquisition costs of the Fairfax Hospital.
[c] For operative prophylaxis, 1 g/2 h for three doses is recommended by Hoechst-Roussel Pharmaceuticals, Inc., in which case the cost of the prophylactic course is $ 28.29.
NA = Investigational drug at printing. No price set at present.

(methicillin, cloxacillin, nafcillin, etc.) exceeding 50% resistance in some centers. Moreover, cephalosporins, may be clinically ineffective against these bacteria despite apparent in vitro sensitivity to them. In fact, methicillin-resistant strains of *Staphylococcus* spp. exhibit cross-resistance to cephalosporins. The standard Kirby-Bauer disc diffusion test may fail to detect this, unless phenotypic expression of methicillin resistance is enhanced by the use of hypertonic media and incubation at lower temperatures.

In hospitals having problems with methicillin-resistant *S. aureus* or *S. epidermidis*, it has been necessary to turn to vancomycin for prophylactic usage [42]. To complicate matters further, certain strains of *S. aureus* exhibit a remarkable tenfold (or greater) increase in their minimum bactericidal concentration (MBC) over their minimum inhibitory concentration (MIC) with respect to penicillins and cephalosporins, a phenomenon called tolerance [67]. Tolerant organisms may be inhibited but not killed by a reasonable serum level of a penicillin or cephalosporin. If staphylococcal tolerance to antibiotics is shown to be a hindrance to the prevention of prosthesis infection, vancomycin may be resorted to even more frequently in the future, as there is no tolerance yet described to this antibiotic.

The 'first-generation' cephalosporins (cephalothin, cefazolin, cephapirin, cephradine) extended the antibacterial spectrum of the semisynthetic penicillins such as nafcillin to include more than *Staphylococcus* and *Streptococcus* spp. They are also effective in the prophylaxis and treatment of infections caused by most *Escherichia coli* and *Klebsiella* species. However, as they have been utilized more and more frequently, they have altered the hospital flora such that many nosocomial infections may be caused by increasingly resistant bacteria such as *Enterobacter*, *Serratia*, and *Pseudomonas* spp. While the newer cephalosporins, penicillins, and related antibiotics possess increased activity against these bacteria, they accordingly lose activity against *Staphylococcus* and *Streptococcus* spp. so that they cannot be considered acceptable prophylactic antibiotics except where cephalothin-resistant gram-negative bacilli are involved. A guide to the use of the older β-lactam antibiotics is shown in table I.

Despite their early promise of efficacy, the newer cephalosporins and penicillins have not fulfilled all expectations of providing a suitable alternative to aminoglycosides for the treatment of cephalothin-resistant bacteria, such as *Enterobacter*, *Serratia*, or *Pseudomonas* spp. These bacteria may develop resistance to the β-lactam antibiotics during therapy. For example, this phenomenon occurred in 16% of patients with *P. aeruginosa* infections treated with piperacillin [24] and 38% treated with moxalactam [59]. At least part of the explanation may be the 'inoculum effect' on the MICs of these bacteria [14]. The inoculum effect is defined as the progressive increase in MICs as the inoculum of bacteria in the broth is increased. This phenomenon is the result of enzymes termed β-lactamases produced by bacteria that inactivate antibiotics. Both *P. aeruginosa* and *Enterobacter* spp. may develop resistance to ceftriaxone [23], but this seems to be less of a problem for both ceftazidime [25] and imipenem [26], especially with regard to *Pseudomonas*. These drugs may be especially useful for the therapy of established infection caused by resistant organisms, but, if they are used frequently for prophylaxis, widespread resistance to these antibiotics may develop within a hospital. The aminocyclitol group of antibiotics - gentamicin, tobramycin, amikacin, and netilmicin - possess exceptional activity against resistant gram-negative bacilli. However, they are toxic to renal function and to hearing and vestibular function, and except when necessary, they are to be avoided in prophylactic situations. If very brief regimens of aminocyclitol antibiotics are utilized prophylactically, they may be associated with less toxicity. However, a clear indication of a cephalothin-resistant organism as a prophylactic target should be identified before they are used. A guide to the use of the new β-lactam antibiotics is shown in table II.

Antibiotic Penetration into Bone

Effective antimicrobial prophylaxis depends on the ability of antibiotics to achieve adequate concentrations at the site of surgery or trauma - in bone, joint, hematoma, or soft tissue. Antibiotics pass through capillaries into the lacunae and canaliculi of bone. From there, they diffuse into the interstitial fluid of the bone matrix of hydroxyapatite crystals and collagen. The diffusion rate of antibiotics into bone is such that normal bone can be saturated within 20–30 min of the intravenous administration of an antibiotic [27]. For that reason, in the prophylaxis of bone surgery, one need administer antibiotics only approximately 30 min prior to the procedure. This slight delay in the penetration into bone from the vascular phase may be due to the physical properties of osseous tissue in somehow inhibiting the penetration of antibiotics [78]. Almost all studies of antibiotic penetration of bone have revealed a tremendous variability in the degree of penetration. The cause of this variability is not known. It is not due to an anatomical or physical barrier [27]. Rather, it may be that metabolic alteration of antibiotics within bone [65] or the assay procedures used for detecting antibiotic concentrations within bone [27] are more likely explanations.

The penetration of cephalosporins into bone has been recently reviewed [27] and the problems associated with the measurement of bone concentrations clearly outlined [66]. In general, the amount of antibiotic in bone is generally lower than the serum, and the concentration in bone increases in proportion to the serum. Most first-generation cephalosporins produce adequate bone levels except for cephalothin. In dogs, cefazolin penetrates readily into normal or osteomyelitic bone [18]. *Schurman* et al. [73] found that in humans the concentration of cefazolin in bone (5.7 μg/g of bone following 1 g i.v.) was above that needed to inhibit *Staphylococcus* spp. and that its penetration was equalled by cephapirin [72]. However, compared to cefazolin or cefoxitin, levels of cephalothin in bone have been observed to decay rather rapidly [66, 71]. *Cunha* et al. [17] administered 1 g each of cefazolin, cephalothin, and cephraradine intravenously and measured bone levels in patients undergoing total hip replacements. Cefazolin achieved the highest concentrations (30 μg/g bone), cephradine second (23 μg/g), and cephalothin the lowest (2.8 μg/g). These unacceptably low cephalothin levels may be enhanced by utilizing an initial loading bolus followed by a constant antibiotic infusion [52]. Similar results were obtained for oxacillin [40] and cephaloridine [39]. However, moderate doses of methicillin (0.5–1 g) did not reliably produce cancellous bone levels in adults while cefazolin did [74]. Vancomycin was found to penetrate both infected and uninfected bone in rabbits. The ratios of serum to bone levels were 7:1 and 10:1, respectively [80]. Third-generation cephalosporins such as moxalactam penetrated bone as well as cefazolin [60].

If the most common error in antibiotic prescription is their overuse, the second most common error is in underdosage of an antibiotic. Prophylaxis, as therapy of established infection, requires full dosages to insure a successful outcome. Tables I and II offer guidelines for the dosages assuming a normal-size adult with nearly normal renal function.

Antibiotic acrylic composites for total joint replacement may be effective prophylactic agents. The acrylic cement, although a hard, brittle material, appears to allow the release of antibiotics along its surface for a relatively long period of time. In a study by *Josefsson* et al.

[38], there were fewer deep infections in patients undergoing total hip replacement who were treated with gentamicin cement than in those with a systemically administered antibiotic. However, there were more superficial infections in the gentamicin cement group. The gentamicin in the cement could not be expected to protect the wound especially from superficial infection by *Streptococcus* species. There have been no reported allergies to the antibiotic-acrylic combination but should such a phenomenon occur, this would be a relatively big problem as the cement cannot easily be removed. There also is some question as to decreased strength of the cement if additional substances are included. Porous coated joint implants are now being utilized that avoid cement altogether.

The efficacy of local antibiotic administration within wounds is controversial. No studies have shown efficacy of irrigation solutions in preventing infection [47, 50]. Tissue concentrations of antibiotic instilled into wounds may be too low to achieve a prophylactic effect on bacteria invading tissue [2]. However, suction drainage devices have been utilized to reduce hematomas postoperatively, and therein probably infections as well.

Indications for Antibiotic Prophylaxis

Open Fractures

There are several situations in which antibiotic prophylaxis may be indicated either because of the degree of wound contamination (open fracture, animal and human bites, or puncture wounds of the foot) or the seriousness of the result of infection (total joint replacement, the insertion of a Harrington rod, and the repair of fractured hips). Of these, open fractures are frequently the dirtiest wounds, being heavily contaminated with bacteria. In addition to a heavy inoculum of bacteria, there is frequently within these wounds ischemic or necrotic tissue which has decreased ability to resist infection. With appropriate debridement, irrigation, and antibiotic prophylaxis, infection can be prevented.

Debridement of wounds requires first of all the removal of foreign bodies and devascularized bone and soft tissue. The wound should then be copiously irrigated with normal saline. The use of antibiotics added to the solution has no further benefit [3, 47]. Internal fixation should not be used initially in dirty open fractures. Rather, stability can be achieved by external fixation utilizing a Hoffman or similar apparatus, or by casting techniques. In cleaner open fractures *Benson* [1] has utilized internal fixation in open fractures without an increase in infection rate. He closed these sorts of wounds primarily, but present teaching [54] suggests that cleaner wounds, as well as dirty wounds, be left open and only closed by delayed primary technique 3–6 days after debridement if the wound is clean at that time.

Delaying wound closure in open fractures for up to 6 days does not increase the risk of infection and may be a more conservative course for segmental open fractures, open fractures with extensive avulsion of soft tissue, and for traumatic amputation. In these situations, infection rates can be as high as 44% [31]. After approximately 1 week's time, resistant gram-negative bacilli such as *P. aeruginosa* and Enterobacter spp. may begin to colonize the wound. Therefore, if there is extensive destruction of soft tissue, the wounds should be covered after 4–6 days by a muscle flap or muscle pedicle graft to protect the exposed bone, and the wound should be closed by skin grafting shortly thereafter.

Determination of the relative contamination of wounds on the basis of gross examination may not always be possible. Wounds that appear clean may have relatively high bacterial counts. To more precisely define conditions in which internal fixation and/or primary wound closure may be considerations, quantitative bacterial cultures may be useful. Using this technique, *Cooney* et al. [13], *Robson and Heggers* [64], and *Benson* [1] all showed that if more than 10^5 organisms per gram of tissue are cultured from a wound, infection will occur in more than 80% of wounds managed by primary closure. However, if the bacterial count is less than 10^5 organisms per gram of tissue, the wounds can be safely closed. Both *Benson* [1] and *Gustilo and Anderson* [31] showed that a relatively clean open fracture may be closed primarily without increasing the risk of infection, provided appropriate antibiotic prophylaxis is employed. *Gustilo and Anderson* [31] showed that a relatively clean open fracture may be closed primarily without increasing the risk of infection, provided appropriate antibiotic prophylaxis is employed. *Gustilo and Anderson* [31] employed the combination of oxacillin and ampicillin for 3 days postoperatively with an infection rate of 2.5%. *Benson* [1] utilized clindamycin or cefazolin for 5 days with a wound infection rate of 6.5%. Neither study had a concurrent control group. How a surgeon may determine prospectively that his patient's wound contains fewer than 10^5 bacteria per gram of tissue is unclear. Unless possibly a gram-stained specimen from the wound be immediately examined, it is risky to employ a primary closure of an open fracture wound when the quantitative bacterial count is not available.

While many have suggested that the use of antibiotics in the setting of open fractures is not prophylactic but rather therapeutic [1, 31, 54–57], open fractures are not initially *infected* but rather heavily *colonized* with bacteria. With appropriate debridement, irrigation, and antibiotic prophylaxis, infection can be prevented. Initial cultures may be positive in more than half of the wounds even before infection is apparent. The most frequent organism cultured is *S. aureus* but many organisms can be present initially [54–56]. Gram-negative bacilli, although less frequent, cause infection in approximately half the cases when they do appear in the initial culture. This fact may reflect their relative resistance to conventional prophylactic agents such as first-generation cephalosporins. When cephalothin-resistant species such as *Enterobacter, Serratia, Aeromonas*, and *P. aeruginosa* are initially cultured from these wounds, an aminocyclitol should be used and the first-generation cephalosporin switched to a third-generation cephalosporin or penicillin to which the organism is sensitive. For *Enterobacter* spp. and *P. aeruginosa*, ticarcillin, mezlocillin, azlocillin, or piperacillin combined with an aminocyclitol such as gentamicin, tobramycin or amikacin, may provide the best protection. *Serratia* and *Aeromonas* spp. may be treated by single therapy with a third-generation cephalosporin such as ceftriaxone, ceftazidime, cefoperazone, cefotaxime, or moxalactam, without utilizing an aminocyclitol, although occasionally a *Serratia* sp. will prove refractory to single therapy with a cephalosporin. Single-drug therapy with a cephalosporin is utilized less frequently for *Enterobacter* spp. and *P. aeruginosa* because of the development of antibiotic resistance that may occur in these organisms during therapy. While newer drugs such as ceftazidime, cefsulodin, or imipenem may prove effective especially for *P. aeruginosa* prophylaxis (or therapy) without the addition of an aminocyclitol, *Enterobacter* spp. have proved to be the more recalcitrant to the new β-lactam antibiotics.

Patzakis et al. [55] utilized cephalothin for 10 days and could reduce the wound infection rate in open fractures from 13.9% when no antibiotics were used to 2.3%. Studies from other centers support these findings [1, 31]. *Patzakis* et al. [54] also utilized cephalothin in prophylaxis of open joint fractures with an infection rate of 2.1%. If displacement was present, open reduction with internal fixation was delayed until 10–14 days later, providing infection was not present at that time. These authors employed primary wound closure and prolonged suction irrigation of open joint fractures especially when there was extensive contamination or tissue damage. However, 14.3% of their patients with initially sterile cultures developed positive cultures postoperatively. The development of nosocomial infection here may have been the result of the prolongation of suction irrigation. Early discontinuation of suction irrigation after 1–2 days is to be recommended.

When cephalothin is utilized frequently within a hospital, cephalothin-resistant gram-negative bacilli may cause nosocomial wound infections. In a hospital with a high incidence of nosocomial infections caused by cephalothin-resistant gram-negative bacilli, the combined use of a cephalosporin and an aminocyclitol has been recommended [53]. If there is a possibility that *Clostridium perfringens* is present within a wound such as occurs with fecal contamination of wounds, penicillin should be utilized in high dosage and any necrotic tissue must be debrided. Hyperbaric oxygen has been recommended but mostly in therapeutic contexts [35]. For penicillin-allergic patients, chloramphenicol may be used. Finally, a patient's tetanus immunization status should be ascertained and tetanus toxoid or tetanus immune globulin administered.

Antibiotics need not be continued longer than 3 days for the prevention of infection of open fractures [31, 53, 57], contrary to previous studies [54, 55] which utilized courses as long as 10 days with no greater efficacy. In patients who received 10-day courses, antibiotic toxicity was directly proportional to the length of antibiotic therapy. 3% of these patients experienced side effects as opposed to only 1% of those who received 3-day courses.

Puncture Wounds of the Foot

When a person steps on a clean nail, a heavy inoculum of *P. aeruginosa* colonizing the inside of the shoe or on the surface of the foot may be driven into the foot resulting in *P. aeruginosa* osteomyelitis [4, 46]. For patients with nail puncture wounds of the feet, thorough debridement and irrigation are indicated, and not infrequently a piece of sock is found within the tissues. Oral cephalosporins are ineffective against *P. aeruginosa.* Only antimicrobial therapy directed against this organism would be expected to provide effective prophylaxis in this situation. At the present time there are only two choices regarding antibiotic prophylaxis. The first is to utilize no drug since no trials have demonstrated a necessity to prescribe prophylactic antibiotics in this setting. The second is to prescribe intravenous or intramuscular aminocyclitols, admitting the patient to the hospital or utilizing an outpatient setting for the parenteral administration of the drug [62]. In the future, another option will be available to provide antibiotic prophylaxis without requiring admission to the hospital. The quinolone class of antibiotics (ciprofloxacin, enoxacin, but not norfloxacin) may provide adequate tissue levels for the treatment of *P. aeruginosa* infections. However, these drugs are still investigational, and efficacy for wound infections is yet to be demonstrated. Oral carbenicillin like norfloxacin does not provide adequate tissue levels.

Patients with diabetes mellitus who suffer puncture wounds of the feet or plantar ulcers may develop infections due to *S. aureus* or polymicrobial infections involving anaerobes. Here, debridement and probably prophylactic antibiotics as well are indicated, although no studies have proven this point.

Animal and Human Bites

Patients who are bitten by animals frequently develop a cellulitis. Although initial cultures may show a variety of anaerobic bacteria in the wounds [30], infections that develop generally are caused by *P. multocida.* This organism is sensitive to penicillin. In penicillin-allergic individuals, tetracycline is a suitable alternative, but cephalosporins are ineffective. While there have been no controlled trials utilizing oral penicillin to prevent infection following animal bites, it may be useful as an adjunct to thorough cleansing of the wound. This is especially true if the joint space or the periosteum has been violated, for *P. multocida* can cause an especially virulent septic arthritis or osteomyelitis.

Human bites are quite different. In this case, the offending organisms that cause cellulitis following a bite are the mouth anaerobes, almost all of which are sensitive to penicillin or clindamycin [30]. Although there are no controlled studies showing their efficacy, severe human bites that violate the joint space or periosteum should probably be prophylaxed with oral penicillin or clindamycin since a human bite introduces a heavy inoculum of bacteria into wounds.

Total Joint Replacement

Infections of total joint replacements have been divided into three categories: (1) Superficial infections - wound infections occurring soon after surgery, not involving the prosthesis; (2) early prosthesis infections - deep infections involving the prosthesis within 1 year postoperatively, and (3) late prosthesis infections - deep infections beyond the first postoperative year. Prosthesis infections tend to be low-grade, subacute infections which are difficult to diagnose, the result of the bacteria seeded at the time of surgery (early and late infections) or of postoperative hematogenous dissemination to the prosthesis (late infections).

To reduce the incidence of early prosthesis infection, *Charnley* pioneered the use of a special operating room environment with special attention to reducing the bacterial contamination of the wound from the air [9, 10, 33]. In his experience, the incidence of late infection also fell parallel to that of early infection, and he felt that late infection was merely due to reactivation of dormant organisms introduced at the time of surgery. This idea was further supported by *Carlsson* et al. [8] extending previous work [22] utilizing perioperative cloxacillin versus no antibiotic in reducing the rate of late (as well as early) infection following total hip replacements from 15.4 to 2%. However, on the basis of anecdotal reports [7, 16, 19, 32, 37, 43, 44, 70, 75] of the infection of total joint replacements by bacteria previously isolated from a blood culture or a distant site of infection, it must be presumed that a portion of late infections may be due to hematogenous seeding. Therefore, late infections probably ought to be excluded from evaluation of perioperative antibiotic prophylaxis, as they may be heterogeneous collections of infections, some seeded intraoperatively and some seeded hematogenously at a later time.

Studies of antibiotic prophylaxis following total joint replacement have revealed efficacy of a variety of different antibiotics. Studies by *Carlsson* et al. [8] and *Ericson* et al. [22] suggested that cloxacillin for 14 days was effective in reducing the infection rate from 17% to 0% in total hip replacement when compared to placebo. One criticism [51] of these studies was that the infection rate of 17% in the placebo group appeared to be quite high. *Schulitz* et al. [69] compared lincomycin for 10 days postoperatively to no antibiotic following total hip replacement, and a significant lowering of deep infection rate to 1% was noted in the lincomycin group compared to 9% for the group receiving no antibiotic. No effect was noted on the rate of occurrence of supeficial infections in the lincomycin group. This study was neither placebo controlled nor blinded [51]. As far as duration of therapy is concerned, *Pollard* et al. [61] obtained an infection rate of 1.3% whether three doses of cephaloridine (for 1 day) or flucloxacillin for 14 days was administered. As in other situations in which prophylactic antibiotics have been shown to be effective in orthopedic surgery, a short course of antibiotics is as effective as a long course.

The use of prophylactic antibiotics in addition to ultraclean air for operating rooms is controversial. *Hill* et al. [34] in a controlled study of cefazolin for 5 days postoperatively showed that infection was significantly greater in the placebo group (3.3%) compared to the antibiotic group (1%). However, when the results were broken down by the type of operating room, operations performed in hypersterile rooms had an infection rate of 1.3 and 0.8% in the treated and placebo groups while those in conventional operating theaters had infection rates of 0.7 and 5.2%, respectively. Only in conventional operating rooms were the differences statistically significant. Infections that did occur in the cefazolin-treated group were cefazolin-resistant ones compared to the placebo group (82 vs. 44%). Antibiotic prophylaxis may provide no additional lowering of the infection rate beyond that provided by ultraclean air.

Lidwell et al. [41] employed whole-body exhaust ventilated suits in operating theaters with ultraclean air reducing infections of total joint replacements to 0.6% as compared to a rate of 1.5% in conventional operating rooms. When all patients were considered together (ultraclean air and conventional operating room patients), the use of an antibiotic reduced the infection rate from 2.3% without an antibiotic to 0.6%. Of those joint replacements performed in conventional operating rooms without antibiotics, 3.4% became infected compared to 0.8% who received antibiotics. In ultraclean operating rooms, the infection rate without antibiotics was 1.2% compared to 0.3% with antibiotics. All results are statistically significant, but the study was not desigend to determine any additional benefit of prophylactic antibiotics in addition to ultraclean air. The use of antibiotics and gentamicin-impregnated cement was done in a nonrandomized fashion, invalidating the results with respect to the benefit of adding antibiotics [51].

Antibiotic-impregnated cement utilized in total joint replacements appears to be effective in reducing prosthesis infections. These infections were significantly reduced in patients who received gentamicin cement (0.4%) compared with those treated with a variety of systemic antibiotics (1.6%). Since this was a multicenter trial and different systemic antibiotics were used in different centers, the significance of these results has been questioned [51]. Furthermore, the gentamicin cement had no effect on superficial infections. Superficial infection was significantly more common in patients receiving gentamicin-impregnated cement (8.3%) versus those treated with systemic antibiotic prophylaxis (5.9%) [38]. Gentamicin-impregnated cement has generally been employed in replacement of a previously infected total joint replacement.

Repair of Hip Fractures (Other Than Total Joint Replacements)

In the prophylaxis of infection following repair of fractured hips, the use of nafcillin for 48 h postoperatively versus placebo was shown by *Boyd* et al. [3] to reduce the wound infection rate from 4.8 to 0.8%. No difference could be demonstrated in the incidence of infected hematomas [51]. A second study by *Burnett* et al. [6] confirmed these results. Cephalothin administered for 24 h prior to and 72 h following surgical repairs of fractured hips reduced infection from 4.7% in the placebo group to 0.7% in the therapeutic group. In those infections that did occur, cephalothin-resistant organisms were frequently identified. In a third study by *Tengve and Kjellander* [77] infection was reduced to 0.8% by utilizing cephalothin and cephalexin for 2 days postoperatively. Unlike the two previous studies, this one was not placebo-controlled.

Elective Orthopedic Surgery

The incidence of infections following elective orthopedic procedures including hip replacement may range from 0.7 to 9% with the highest rate occurring in hip fracture repairs involving the insertion of prosthetic material. *Pavel* et al. [58] showed that the wound infection rate for clean orthopedic surgery could be reduced by cephaloridine from 5% in those receiving placebo to 2.8%. Although this study was double-blinded and placebo-controlled, there was some question as to whether a selection bias may have been introduced since 887 patients received antibiotic while only 704 received placebo [51]. *Fogelberg* et al. [28] reported similar results by combining figures of the prophylaxis of infection following mold arthroplasty and spine fusion. They showed an overall reduction in wound infection rate from 8.9% in those receiving no antibiotic to 1.7% in a group receiving penicillin. This study has been criticized on two grounds [2]. First of all, the results of two different procedures were combined. Secondly, when the results were taken separately, beneficial effects of antibiotic prophylaxis were seen only for spine fusions and not for mold arthroplasties. For spine fusions alone, the infection rate was reduced from 5.5% for controls (no antibiotic) to 0% in the penicillin group. However, these groups were not large enough to obtain statistical significance. Finally, penicillin is no longer the drug of choice in preventing *S. aureus* infections as 90% of these organisms are now resistant to this antibiotic.

Conclusions

There are two general indications for antibiotic prophylaxis. The first, epitomized by the open fracture, is a heavily contaminated wound which is likely to become infected. The second situation, of which the total joint replacement is a good example, is a wound which may have a low incidence of infection, but, if it becomes infected, the results are a calamity. In these situations, prophylactic antibiotics appear to be useful providing (1) they are administered at the time of maximal bacterial contamination of the wound, (2) they penetrate the wound or bone effectively, and (3) they are active against the bacteria expected to cause infection within the wound.

Prophylactic antibiotics have been shown to be effective in total joint replacement, in hip fracture repairs, and in the management of dirty wounds including open fractures. There are no good studies concerning their use in nail puncture wounds of the foot and in human and animal bites, but it is anticipated that antibiotic prophylaxis trials might show some benefit here. Controversy surrounds the use of antibiotics to prevent infection following elective orthopedic procedures other than total joint replacement or hip fracture repair.

The choice of an antibiotic for prophylaxis depends on the bacteria likely to be present within the wound. For total joint replacement or for repair of a fractured hip, cefazolin seems to be a good choice in view of its good activity against *Staphylococcus* and *Streptococcus* spp., its good bone penetration, its favorable pharmacokinetics allowing three times daily administration, its low incidence of adverse drug reactions, and its low cost. For severe penicillin or cephalosporin allergy, vancomycin is the drug of choice. However, it is more toxic (to the hearing and the kidneys) and more expensive. With the use of shorter courses of antibiotics (possibly a single dose administered preoperatively), the cost and potential side effects of antibiotic prophylaxis can be further reduced, to make prophylactic antibiotics even more cost-effective in economic as well as in human terms.

Acknowledgements

The time, effort, and constructive suggestions of *Jeffrey Malka*, MD, and *Peter Bruno*, MD, in reviewing this manuscript from the orthopedic surgeon's viewpoint is gratefully acknowledged. *Donald M. Poretz*, MD, and *Robin I. Goldenberg*, MD, critically reviewed it from the infectious diseases physician's perspective.

References

1 Benson, D.R.; Riggins, R.S.; Lawrence, R.M.; Hoeprich, P.D.; Huston, A.C.; Harrison, J.A.: Treatment of open fractures: a prospective study. J. Trauma *23:* 25–30 (1983).
2 Boyd, R.J.: Orthopedic surgery. J. Bone Jt Surg. *70:* suppl. 1, pp. 48–50 (1977).
3 Boyd, R.J.; Burke, J.F.; Colton, T.C.: A double-blind clinical trial of prophylactic antibiotics in hip fracture patients. J. Bone Jt Surg. *55:* 1251–1259 (1973).
4 Brand, R.A.; Black, H.: Pseudomonas osteomyelitis following puncture wounds in children. J. Bone Jt Surg. *56–A:* 1637–1642 (1974).
5 Burke, J.F.: The effective period of preventive antibiotic action in experimental incisions and dermal lesions. Surgery *50:* 161–168 (1961).
6 Burnett, J.W.; Gustilo, R.B.; Williams, D.N.; Kind, A.C.: Prophylactic antibiotics in hip fractures. A double-blind, prospective study. J. Bone Jt Surg. *62–A:* 457–462 (1980).
7 Burton, D.S.; Schurman, D.J.: Case report of delayed infection of bilateral total hip arthroplasties of probable hematogenous origin. J. Bone Jt Surg. *57–A:* 1004–1005 (1975).
8 Carlsson, A.S.; Lidgren, L.; Lindberg, L.: Prophylactic antibiotics against early and late deep infections after total hip replacements. Acta orthop. scand. *48:* 405–410 (1977).
9 Charnley, J.: Postoperative infection after total hip replacement with special reference to air contamination in the operating room. Clin. Orthop. *87:* 167–187 (1972).

10 Charnley, J.; Cupic, Z.: The nine- and ten-year results of the low-friction arthroplasty of the hip. Clin. Orthop. *95:* 9–25 (1973).
11 Charnley, J.; Eftekhar, N.: Postoperative infection in total prosthetic replacement arthroplasty of the hip joint with special reference to the bacterial content of the air of the operating room. Br. J. Surg. *56:* 641–649 (1969).
12 Collis, D.K.; Steinhaus, K.: Total hip replacement without deep infection in a standard operating room. J. Bone Jt Surg. *58-A:* 446–450 (1976).
13 Cooney, W.P.; Fitzgerald, R.H.; Dobyns, J.H.; Washington, J.A.: Quantitative wound cultures in upper extremity trauma. J. Trauma *22:* 112–117 (1982).
14 Corrado, M.L.; Landesman, S.H.; Cherubin, C.E.: Influence of inoculum size on activity of cefoperazone, cefotaxime, moxalactam, piperacillin, and N-formimidoyl thienamycin (MK0787) against *Pseudomonas aeruginosa.* Antimicrob. Agents Chemother. *18:* 893–896 (1980).
15 Coventry, M.B.; Beckenbaugh, R.D.; Nolan, D.R.; Ilstrup, D.M.: 2,012 total hip arthroplasties: a study of postoperative course and early infections. J. Bone Jt Surg. *56-A:* 278–284 (1974).
16 Creuss, R.L.; Bickel, W.S.; Kessler, K.L.C. von: Infections in total hips secondary to a primary source elsewhere. Clin. Orthop. *106:* 99–101 (1975).
17 Cunha, B.A.; Gossling, H.R.; Pasternak, H.S.; Nightingale, C.H.; Quintiliani, R.: The penetration characteristics of cefazolin, cephalothin, and cephradine into bone in patients undergoing total hip replacement. J. Bone Jt Surg. *59-A:* 856–859 (1977).
18 Daly, R.C.; Fitzgerald, R.H.; Washington, J.A.: Penetration of cefazolin into normal and osteomyelitic canine cortical bone. Antimicrob. Agents Chemother. *22:* 461–469 (1982).
19 Downes, E.M.: Late infection after total hip replacement. J. Bone Jt Surg. *59-B:* 42–44 (1977).
20 Elek, S.D.: Experimental staphylococcal infections in the skin of man. Ann. N.Y. Acad. Sci. *65:* 85–90 (1956–1957).
21 Elek, S.D.; Conen, P.E.: The virulence of *Staphylococcus pyogenes* for man: a study of the problem of wound infections. Br. J. exp. Pathol. *38:* 573–588 (1957).
22 Ericson, C.; Lidgren, L.; Lindberg, L.: Cloxacillin in the prophylaxis of postoperative infections of the hip. J. Bone Jt Surg. *55-A:* 808–813 (1973).
23 Eron, L.J.; Park, C.H.; Goldenberg, R.I.; Poretz, D.M.: Ceftriaxone therapy of bone and soft tissue infections in hospital and outpatient settings. Antimicrob. Agents Chemother. *23:* 731–737 (1983).
24 Eron, L.J.; Goldenberg, R.I.; Poretz, D.M.; Park, C.H.: Piperacillin therapy for *Pseudomonas* infections. Sth. med. J. *76:* 859–862 (1983).
25 Eron, L.J.; Goldenberg, R.I.; Park, C.H.; Poretz, D.M.: Ceftazidime therapy of serious bacterial infections. Antimicrob. Agents Chemother. *23:* 236–241 (1983).
26 Eron, L.J.; Hixon, D.L.; Park, C.H.; Goldenberg, R.I.; Poretz, D.M.: Imipenem versus moxalactam in the treatment of serious infections. Antimicrob. Agents Chemother. *24:* 841–846 (1983).
27 Fitzgerald, R.H.; Thompson, R.L.: Cephalosporin antibiotics in the prevention and treatment of musculoskeletal sepsis. J. Bone Jt Surg. *65-A:* 1201–1205 (1983).
28 Fogelberg, E.V.; Zitzmann, E.K.; Stinchfield, F.E.: Prophylactic penicillin in orthopedic surgery. J. Bone Jt Surg. *52-A:* 95–98 (1970).

29 Goldner, J.L.; Allen, B.L.: Ultraviolet light in orthopedic operating rooms at Duke University. Clin. Orthop. *96:* 195-205 (1973).

30 Goldstein, E.J.C.; Citron, D.M.; Wield, B.; Blachman, U.; Sutter, V.L.; Miller, T.A.; Finegold, S.M.: Bacteriology of human and animal bite wounds. J. clin. Microbiol. *8:* 667-672 (1978).

31 Gustilo, R.B.; Anderson, J.T.: Prevention of infection in the treatment of one thousand and twenty-five open fractures of long bones. J. Bone Jt Surg. *58-A:* 453-458 (1976).

32 Hall, A.J.: Late infection about a total knee prosthesis. J. Bone Jt Surg. *56-B:* 144-147 (1974).

33 Hicks, J.H.: The relationship between metal and infection. Proc. R. Soc. Med. *50:* 842-844 (1957).

34 Hill, C.; Flamant, R.; Mazas, F.; Evrard, J.: Prophylactic cefazolin versus placebo in total hip replacement. Report of a multicenter double-blind randomised trial. Lancet *i:* 795-797 (1981).

35 Hitchcock, C.R.; Demello, F.J.; Haglin, J.J.: Gangrene infection: new approaches to an old disease. Surg. Clins N. Am. *55:* 1403-1410 (1975).

36 Howe, C.W.; Marston, A.T.: A study on sources of postoperative staphylococcal infection. Surgery Gynec. Obstet. *115:* 266-275 (1962).

37 Jacobsen, P.L.; Murray, W.: Prophylactic coverage of dental patients with artificial joints: a retrospective analysis of thirty-three infections in hip prostheses. Oral Surg. *50:* 130-133 (1980).

38 Josefsson, G.; Lindberg, L.; Wiklander, B.: Systemic antibiotics and gentamicin-containing bone cement in the prophylaxis of perioperative infections in total hip arthroplasty. Clin. Orthop. *159:* 194-200 (1981).

39 Kanyuck, D.O.; Welles, J.S.; Emerson, J.L.; Anderson, R.C.: The penetration of cephalosporin antibiotics into bone. Proc. Soc. exp. Biol. Med. *136:* 997-999 (1971).

40 Kolczun, M.C.; Nelson, C.L.; McHenry, M.C.; Govan, J.L.; Pinovich, P.: Antibiotic concentrations in human bone. J. Bone Jt Surg. *56-A:* 305-309 (1974).

41 Lidwell, O.M.; Lowbury, E.J.L.; Whyte, W.; Blowers, R.; Stanley, S.J.; Lowe, D.: Effect of ultraclean air in operating rooms on deep sepsis in the joint after total hip or knee replacement: a randomised study. Br. med. J. *285:* 10-14 (1982).

42 Lowy, F.D.; Hamner, S.M.: *Staphylococcus epidermidis* infections. Ann. intern. Med. *99:* 834-839 (1983).

43 Mallory, T.H.: Sepsis in total hip replacement following pneumococcal pneumonia. J. Bone Jt Surg. *55-A:* 1753-1754 (1973).

44 Marmor, L.; Berkus, D.: Hematogenous infection of total knee implants. Surgery *83:* 291-292 (1978).

45 Miles, A.A.; Miles, E.M.; Burke, J.: The value and duration of defence reactions of the skin to the primary lodgement of bacteria. Br. J. exp. Path. *38:* 79-96 (1957).

46 Miller, E.H.; Semian, D.W.: Gram-negative osteomyelitis following puncture wounds of the foot. J. Bone Jt Surg. *57-A:* 535-537 (1975).

47 Nachamie, B.; Siffert, R.S.; Bryer, M.S.: A study of neomycin installation into orthopedic surgical wounds. J. Am. med. Ass. *204:* 139-141 (1968).

48 Nelson, J.P.; Glassburn, A.R.; Talbott, R.D.; McElhinney, J.P.: Clean room operating rooms. Clin. Orthop. *96:* 179-187 (1973).

49 Nelson, C.L.; Green, T.G.; Porter, R.A.; Warren, R.D.: One day versus seven days of preventive antibiotic therapy in orthopedic surgery. Clin. Orthop. *176:* 258–263 (1983).
50 Norden, C.W.: Antibiotic prophylaxis in orthopedic surgery. Clin. Orthop. *114:* 203–206 (1976).
51 Norden, C.W.: A critical review of antibiotic prophylaxis in orthopedic surgery. Rev. infect. Dis. *5:* 928–932 (1983).
52 Patel, D.; Moellering, R.C.; Thrasker, K.; Fahmy, N.R.; Harris, W.H.: The effect of hypotensive anesthesia and cephalothin concentration in bone and muscle of patients undergoing total hip replacement. J. Bone Jt Surg. *61–A:* 531–538 (1979).
53 Patzakis, M.: Management of open fractures and complications; in Frankel, Instructional course lectures, vol. 31, pp. 62–64 (Mosby, St. Louis 1982).
54 Patzakis, M.J.; Dorr, L.D.; Ivler, D.; Moore, T.M.; Harvey, J.P.: The early management of open joint injuries. J. Bone Jt Surg. *57–A:* 1065-1071 (1975).
55 Patzakis, M.J.; Harvey, J.P.; Ivler, D.: The role of antibiotics in the management of open fractures. J. Bone Jt. Surg. *56–A:* 532–541 (1974).
56 Patzakis, M.J.; Ivler, D.: Antibiotic and bacteriologic considerations in open fractures. Sth. med. J. *70:* suppl., 1, pp. 46–48 (1977).
57 Patzakis, M.J.; Wilkins, J.; Moore, T.M.: Considerations in reducing the infection rate in open tibial fractures. Clin. Orthop. *178:* 36–41 (1983).
58 Pavel, A.; Smith, R.L.; Ballard, A.; Larson, I.J.: Prophylactic antibiotics in clean orthopedic surgery. J. Bone Jt Surg. *56–A:* 777–782 (1974).
59 Platt, R.; Ehrlich, S.L.; Afarian, J.; O'Brien, T.F.; Pennington, J.E.; Kass, E.H.: Moxalactam therapy of infections caused by cephalothin-resistant bacteria: influence of serum inhibitory activity on clinical response and acquisition of antibiotic resistance during therapy. Antimicrob. Agents Chemother. *20:* 351–355 (1981).
60 Polk, R.; Hume, A.; Kline, B.J.; Cardea, J.: Penetration of moxalactam and cefazolin into bone following simultaneous bolus or infusion. J. clin. Orthop. *177:* 216–221 (1983).
61 Pollard, J.P.; Hughes, S.P.F.; Scott, J.E.; Evans, M.J.; Benson, M.K.D.: Antibiotic prophylaxis in total hip replacement. Br. med. J. *i:* 707–709 (1979).
62 Poretz, D.M.; Eron, L.J.; Goldenberg, R.I.; Gilbert, A.F.; Rising, J.; Sparks, S.; Horn, C.E.: Intravenous antibiotic therapy in an outpatient setting. J. Am. med. Ass. *248:* 336–339 (1982).
63 Robson, M.C.; Krizek, T.J.; Heggers, J.P.: Biology of surgical infection. Curr. Probl. Surg. *March:* 1–62 (1973).
64 Robson, M.C.; Heggers, J.P.: Bacterial quantification of open wounds. Military Med. *134:* 19–24 (1969).
65 Rosdahl, V.T.; Sorensen, T.S.; Colding, H.: Determination of antibiotic concentrations in bone. J. Antimicrob. Chemother. *5:* 275–280 (1979).
66 Rosenfeld, M.B.; Campos, J.; Ratzan, K.R.; Uredo, I.: Chemoprophylaxis with cefoxitin and cephalothin in orthopedic surgery: a comparison. Antimicrob. Agents. Chemother. *19:* 826–830 (1981).
67 Sabbath, L.D.; Laverdiere, M.; Wheeler, N.; Blazevic, D.; Wilkinson, B.J.: A new type of penicillin resistance of *Staphylococcus aureus.* Lancet *i:* 443–447 (1977).
68 Salvatti, E.A.; Robinson, R.P.; Zeno, Z.M.; Koslin, B.L.; Brause, B.D.; Wilson,

P.D.: Infection rates after 3175 total hip and total knee replacements performed with and without a horizontal unidirectional filtered air-flow system. J. Bone Jt Surg. *64-A:* 525-535 (1982).

69 Schulitz, K.P.; Winkelmann, W.; Schoening, B.: The prophylactic use of antibiotics in alloarthroplasty of the hip joint for coxarthrosis. Arch Orthop. Trauma *96:* 79-82 (1980).

70 Schurman, D.J.; Aptekar, R.G.; Burton, D.S.: Infection in total knee joint replacement secondary to tooth abscess. West J. Med. *125:* 226-227 (1976).

71 Schurman, D.J.; Burton, D.S.; Kajiyama, G.: Cefoxitin antibiotic concentration in bone and synovial fluid. Clin. Orthop. *168:* 64-68 (1982).

72 Schurman, D.J.; Burton, D.S.; Kajiyama, G.; Moser, K.; Nagel, D.A.: Sodium cephapirin disposition and distribution into human bone. Curr. Ther. Res. *20:* 194-203 (1976).

73 Schurman, D.J.; Hirshman, H.P.; Kajiyama, G.; Moser, K.; Burton, D.S.: Cefazolin concentrations in bone and synovial fluid. J. Bone Jt Surg. *60-A:* 359-362 (1978).

74 Sorensen, T.S.; Colding, H.; Schroeder, E.; Rosdahl, V.T.: The penetration of cefazolin, erythromycin, and methicillin into human bone tissue. Acta orthop. scand. *49:* 549-553 (1978).

75 Stinchfield, F.E.; Bigliani, L.U.; Neu, H.C.; Goss, T.P.; Foster, C.: Late hematogenous infection of total joint replacement. J. Bone Jt. Surg. *62-A:* 1345-1350 (1980).

76 Taylor, F.W.: An experimental evaluation of operative wound irrigation. Surgery Gynec. Obstet. *113:* 465-470 (1961).

77 Tengve, B.; Kjellander, J.: Antibiotic prophylaxis in operations on trochanteric femoral fractures. J. Bone Jt Surg. *60-A:* 97-99 (1978).

78 Verwey, W.F.; Williams, H.R.; Kaslow, C.: Penetration of chemotherapeutic agents into tissues. Antimicrob. Agents Chemother. *1965:* 1016-1024 (1966).

79 Wenzel, R.P.: The emergence of methicillin-resistant *Staphylococcus aureus.* Ann. intern. Med. *97:* 440-441 (1982).

80 Wilson, K.J.; Mader, J.T.: Concentrations of vancomycin in bone and serum of normal rabbits and those with osteomyelitis. Antimicrob. Agents Chemother. *25:* 140-141 (1984).

L.J. Eron, MD, FACP, Division of Infectious Diseases, The Fairfax Hospital, Falls Church, VA 22046 (USA)

Antibiot. Chemother., vol. 33, pp. 165–183 (Karger, Basel 1985)

Perioperative Prevention of Infection in Neurosurgery

D. Voth

Neurochirurgische Klinik und Poliklinik, Johannes Gutenberg-Universität, Mainz, BRD

Introduction

The special clinical features of neurosurgery are the reason why, on the one hand it shares the problems of infection with a whole range of other operative specialities and, on the other hand, has its own particular problems [44, 45].

The surgery of peripheral nerves shares the risks of operations on the soft parts of the extremities and interventions on the vertebral column include the risks of orthopedics, and, finally, the numerous compound injuries correspond to those injuries which are cared for by accident surgery [39, 50]. The high morbidity in clinical conditions which are treatable by shunt procedures with ventriculo-atrial and ventriculoperitoneal systems, provides the risks which develop as a result of implanted synthetic materials [3, 4, 7, 8, 10].

More specific are the risks of infections of the skull cavity, including the central nervous system, in the form of meningitis or brain abscess. Further related problems are the cerebrospinal fluid (CSF) fistulas, which for many years have been the reason for a really futile, and under certain circumstances even dangerous, 'cover' with antibiotics.

In the following, we will first take general note of the dangers of infection and its prophylaxis in order to be able to discuss particular aspects and the practical management of the prophylaxis [5, 43, 48].

General Comments on the Dangers of Infection

In relation to other specialities, we distinguish the following procedures in regard to the potential degrees of contamination:

(1) Strictly aseptic procedures: These are clean, nontraumatic operation wounds, with planned incisions and primary wound healing. Among these are intracranial operations for arterial aneurysms or A-V malformations, intracerebral and extracerebral tumors, and operations on the vertebral column and spinal canal, with or without opening of the dura.

(2) Partially aseptic procedures: Here we are dealing with potentially contaminated wounds, as perhaps after opening of the frontal sinus during a craniotomy, with infections close to the operation field.

(3) Definitely contaminated wounds: These exist with all open injuries, as well as with operations in infected regions of the body. The resection of a brain abscess constitutes a special case.

Violations of the antisepsis and further risk factors such as higher age, cachexia, existing infectious disease, and metabolic disturbances (diabetes mellitus, cirrhosis of the liver, azotemia, etc.) can be the occasion, on account of the danger of contamination, for reclassifying the planned procedure possibly from group 1 to group 2.

Specific to the speciality are, in addition, the following conditions:

(a) Interventions with implantation of synthetic materials which are liable to produce infection, such as shunt operations in cases of hydrocephalus.

(b) Operations in patients with impaired resistance, where in our speciality there has very frequently been immunosuppression as a result of high doses of dexamethasone, and also in patients after cytostatic therapy with nitrosourea derivatives.

Even in strictly aseptic procedures these two groups form a category particularly at risk, as regards infection.

Perioperative prophylaxis has its particular status in neurosurgery due to the fact that infections for instance of the skull contents have immediately fatal consequences and thus the patients are put at risk in a way that does not exist in all other operative specialities.

Factors which Favor Disturbances of Wound Healing

The problem of wound healing is not confined only to the abovementioned factors. Apart from the dangers of contamination of, at times, planned procedures, further factors play a big role.

These may be briefly mentioned: duration of operation; timing of the operations and the amount of use of the operation room; faults in asepsis and antisepsis; unfavorable technical operative details, such as excessive use of coagulation, burying of a lot of sutures and other foreign material.

Thus, some authors describe an increase in the risk of infection, with increasing duration of use of the operation room. Nevertheless, one must distinguish here between the lengthy use during a single operation and between a multiple change of patients with their transfer, increased frequency of preparation, and more frequent passage of personnel back and forth through the doors of the operating room. While in the last instance the risks of contamination certainly rise this does not apply with the same probability to the occasionally very long-lasting microsurgical procedures, for instance, in the posterior fossa. In any case in our speciality one cannot guard against an increase in wound infection with the duration of the operation.

Suspected or more certain violations against asepsis can occur in the operative procedures. Needless to say perioperative prophylaxis cannot be a substitute for an easy-going attitude to asepsis. On the other hand, it would be fatal if the perpetrator of an offence against asepsis kept quiet about it and the operation team were not informed. The safeguarding of a meticulous asepsis, a corresponding discipline and, at the same time, honesty in the case of a violation, should be the golden rule for behavior.

The epidemiology of surgical wound infection is not unimportant when considering the indications for prophylaxis [40]. Here we have noticed a fall in the infections due to a single organism and an increase in mixed infections, although the former, of course, still makes up more than a half of all cases. Just as striking is the change of the spectrum of the pathogens. While there is still a decrease in frequency of the gram-negative organisms such as *Escherichia coli, Klebsiella, Enterobacter, Proteus* spp., *Pseudomonas* and the groups of the more rare gram-negative bacteria, the infections with gram-positive organisms, above all the *Staphylococci* and *Bacteroides* are increasing.

In contrast to the state of affairs in abdominal surgery, infections with a single organism are, of course, much more frequent in neurosurgical patients. The pattern of pathogens can exhibit differences within the speciality in individual clinics according to the habits and peculiarities of the local customs of antibiotic treatment at any one time.

Finally, it should be stated that the care of the wounds and the technique of dressings are undoubtedly factors which influence the incidence of infection. The use of open wound drainage systems is obsolete, but even with the closed systems with vacuum bottles there are marked differences. Not all systems are absolutely definitely sterile or remain so. Here, practical experience has shown that in the manufacture of sterile systems with vacuum bottles definite errors can occur and are identifiable.

That wound dressings should be changed only with sterile gloves, goes without saying. In addition, the technique of suturing is of importance, with possibly too thick buried subcutaneous sutures which affect the blood supply and impair the circulation in the wound edges. These should be avoided.

These comments show that a wound infection can have many causes, but at the same time a not insignificant number of them are caused by factors which the surgeon is able to influence. Here we must start with the prophylaxis of wound infection and not with recourse to antibiotics!

General Discussion on Perioperative Prophylaxis

It is certainly not superfluous to stress that the instillation of antibiotics into a wound is not prophylaxis [29], but in the majority of cases a pointless undertaking and in unfavorable cases is rather dangerous on acount of the risk of sensitisation. Local antibiotic treatment is only justified in quite special situations and with strict indications. Equally obsolete is oral administration. It is quite impractical on account of the fluctuating conditions of absorption and the uncertainties of serum and tissue levels. The only route for perioperative prophylaxis is, as a rule, by parenteral administration.

It can be considered as definite, that a preoperative prophylaxis before the start of an operation has to provide for an adequate tissue level and therefore has to be given at least 1 h pre-operatively, as a rule before the induction of the anesthetic [2, 7]. An antibiotic course which is only given in the afternoon or evening of the operation day, or is even started later, is absurd.

Also, we may regard it as proven that a continuation of the prophylaxis for more than 24 h is inappropriate and futile. In the majority of cases a period of 12 h should be completely adequate. More recent studies substantiate incidentally the completely adequate effect of a single dose pre-operatively, as 'single-dose prophylaxis'.

Nevertheless, it is surprising how few indications have been verified by controlled studies! In not a few situations the neurosurgeon can merely fall back on comparable findings from other specialities [6, 9, 17, 18, 27, 35].

Thus, it is only sensible to undertake a perioperative prophylaxis in neurosurgery if the local conditions are taken into account, as well as the currently accepted general criteria, namely the spectrum of the pathogens and the individual infection rate of each intervention. This, however, requires the neurosurgeon to take care that the relevant date are available to him. For example, in our clinic we obtain the figures monthly from the institute of microbiology so that we can be aware of the pattern of the pathogens in the tests which we have taken, analyzed according to the test material and the organisms.

Thus, for instance in January 1983 the organisms found in the urine tests from our patients showed the following types: *E. coli* 17.1%, *Streptococcus faecalis* 13.7%, *Pseudomonas* sp. 13.7%, *Staphylococcus epidermidis* and *Serratia liq.* each 10.3%. In material from wounds about 60% *Staphylococcus aureus* and *S. epidermidis*, and about 40% *S. faecalis* were found. From the air passages (tracheal swabs, etc.) the commonest were *S. aureus* at 20.4% and *E. coli* with 13.6%. In the total material from all tests (urinary tract, intestinal tract, air passages, blood, CSF, material from wounds) *S. faecalis* was placed first with 19.7%, followed by *S. aureus* with 17.2% and *E. coli* with 13.5%. It goes without saying that these rates are less significant than many of the findings in the individual tests, but they allow one to draw conclusions about the range of pathogens at risk.

Besides the information on the relevant range of pathogens, classified from the various tests, the neurosurgeon, however, requires further information about the current levels of resistance. There is available for us an exact description of the resistance to about 40 antibiotics of all the identified organisms. Although these data are certainly similar to the facts from other neurosurgical clinics, it is my impression that the particular data about the relevant local situation is of considerable significance. Thus, our data for the same month, January 1983 show for *S. aureus* a resistance to penicillin G and ampicillin of around 75%, to the ureidopenicillins, mezlocillin and azlocillin, of 41 and 50%, re-

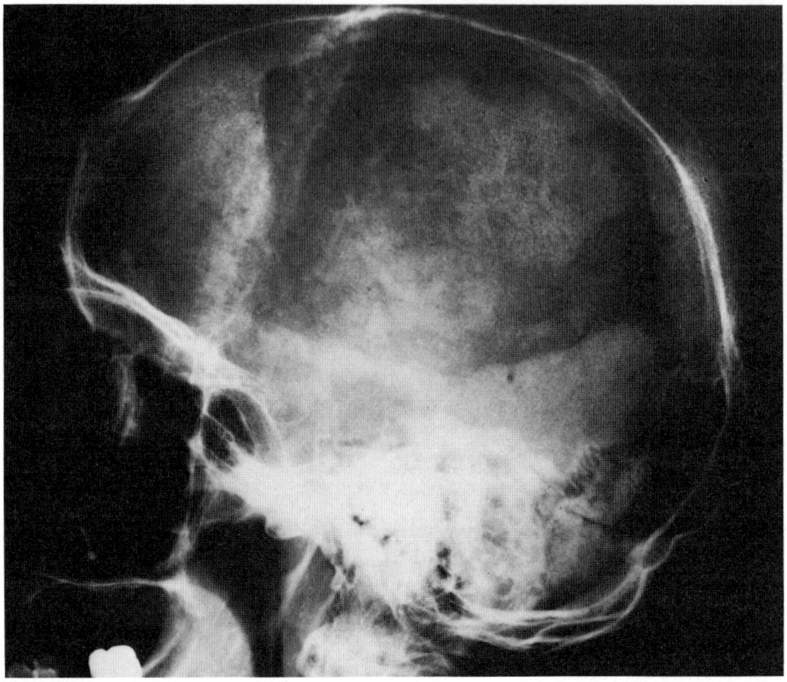

Fig. 1. Osteomyelitis of the bone flap after a left-sided frontoparietal craniotomy in a 43-year-old woman. Not all these lesions are caused by a bacterial infection; they can be a manifestation of a 'sterile' destruction of the skull bones.

spectively, and with regard to oxacillin of only 7%. It is obvious that these results must be taken into consideration when choosing an antibiotic in cases of perioperative prophylaxis [11].

Special Prophylaxis in Neurosurgery

Strictly Aseptic Operations

This group involves operations on the skull and the vertebral column, which take place after adequate preparation time, show no primary risks of infection and are carried out under strictly aseptic conditions. The diagnostic groups include intrinsic and extracerebral intracranial tumors, malformations, and intracerebral and extracerebral hematomas. In the vertebral column we must mention operations on prolapsed intervertebral discs and likewise on spinal tumors.

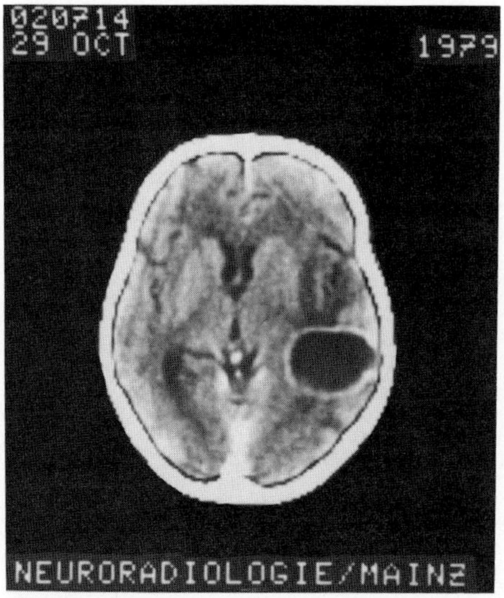

Fig. 2. Computer tomographic picture of a right temporoparietal brain abscess in a 29-year-old man. There is still evidence of perifocal edema. After giving contrast medium there is a clearly defined outlining of the contours of the abscess.

The incidence of infection as shown in the results of individual clinics, shows only slight differences. For operations on the skull one may reckon on infection in about 3–5% of cases; however, in some cases these figures are considerably lower. I can see here primarily no indication for a perioperative prophylaxis.

There is a relative indication if further factors appear, such as advanced age or poor condition of the patient. However, these cannot be regarded as valid for the duration of the operation.

A special problem is osteomyelitis of the bone flap (fig. 1) which is more frequent than an infection in the subdural space. Nevertheless, these changes in the bone flap are more the expression of a sterile bony absorption and only to a certain extent a bacterial infection, which, without exception, starts at the time of the operation. The frequency of the complication, however, is such that any antibiotic prophylaxis is not justified.

Operations on brain abscesses (fig. 2) constitute a special case. With these, the operative approach is strictly aseptic, but the target of the operation is potentially highly infectious. It has been shown in

Table I. Mortality of brain abscesses in the acute and chronic stages, in relation to the various methods of treatment [data from ref. 49]

Treatment	Chronic abscess %	Acute abscess %	Total n	Total mortality, %
Antibiotics	100	50	3	66.6
Antibiotics + operation	29.7 (n = 37)	88.8 (n = 9)	46	41.3
Antibiotics + dexamethasone	25 (n = 4)	12.5 (n = 9)	13	23.1
Antibiotics + dexamethasone + operation	10 (n = 30)	46.7 (n = 15)	45	22.2

these cases that operating in the acute stage is extremely risky. The maxim which still holds good today in all cases is to first try to treat the abscess by conservative measures (dexamethasone + antibiotics), until it has disappeared on the CT, or until no further tendency to regression is apparent. The operation can then be performed, if it still appears necessary, in the chronic stage after formation of a glial capsule. In general, an operation in the acute stage is dangerous [49] and should be avoided if at all possible (table I). If the removal of the residual abscess is then planned the procedure must take place under antibiotic prophylaxis. In some cases the organism involved is already known from an earlier puncture, so that a specific attack is possible. In these cases it is worth taking care that the blood level is high enough and, in addition, that the tissue level in the brain is also high as the blood brain barrier in the region of the abscess is no longer intact. Antibiotics which will cross into the CSF should, nevertheless, be preferred.

In these cases it seems that a prophylaxis over 12 h up to a maximum of 24 h is justifiable as the height of the attainable tissue level, in comparison with the other tissues, cannot be accurately predicted.

Although we must consider that the removal of a brain abscess must be grouped with operations in a probably contaminated field there exist a whole range of unusual features. Above all, there is the fact that after prolonged and adequate conservative treatment the abscess has a tough glial capsule and if it remains unopened the whole proce-

Table II. Survey of the inflammatory complications after operations on lumbar disc lesions; the data from Giessen are taken from *Schepelmann* et al. [38], the figures from the Mainz clinic were published by *Meinig* et al. [31]

1 Disturbances of wound healing (not only infections)	7.6%	Mainz 1972–1982 18.8%, Giessen
2 Spondylodiscitis	1.03%	Mainz, 1970–1980 0.15%, Mainz 1956–1970 1.5%, Giessen
3 Phlegmon (subfascial)	0.5%	

dure can remain completely aseptic. However, if the abscess is ruptured this situation becomes fundamentally changed. In principle, however, one should reckon on this complication occurring and consider that prophylaxis is indicated.

Operations on the spine, possibly for prolapsed intervertebral discs or for tumors, should be regarded basically as strictly aseptic. This holds good for all types of intervention from flavectomy, laminectomy, hemi-laminectomy and microsurgical approaches, right up to the procedures for anterior fusion in the cervical region [23]. Nevertheless, the incidence of infection is not small, as is shown in table II. In general, we find that disturbances of wound healing caused by infection [38] are about 7.6%, although in other publications figures up to about 18.8% are given. These figures are very high although to some extent probably clinical and also other insignificant events are concealed. The serious infections are still rare, such as the sub-fascial infection occurring possibly after a laminectomy (fig. 3). Its frequency is without exception under 1%, so that there is no indication for prophylaxis.

A special complication is postoperative spondylodiscitis (fig. 4). Its frequency is without exception given as around 1%. Here, also, not all observations of a spondylodiscitis may be of the same significance with a bacterial infection as the cause, as a 'sterile' type of course is also well known. The X-ray picture is typical (fig. 4) as also is the clinical course. Its frequency does not justify a general use of antibiotic prophylaxis. In our material the frequency of spondylodiscitis during the period since 1975 amounted to 1.03%, while earlier (1955–1975) it had been around 0.15%. The cause of this increase has not so far been determined [31].

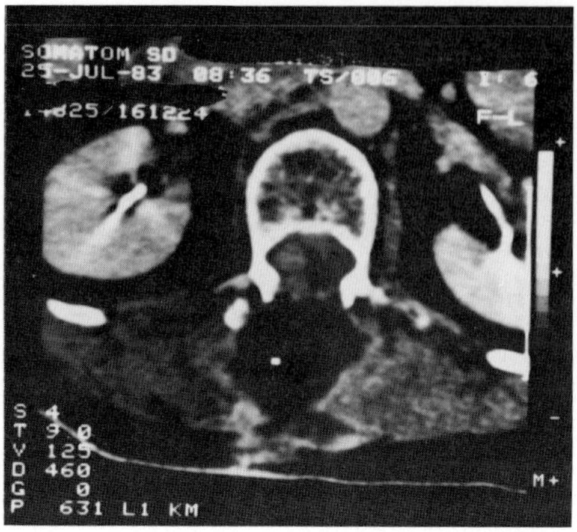

a

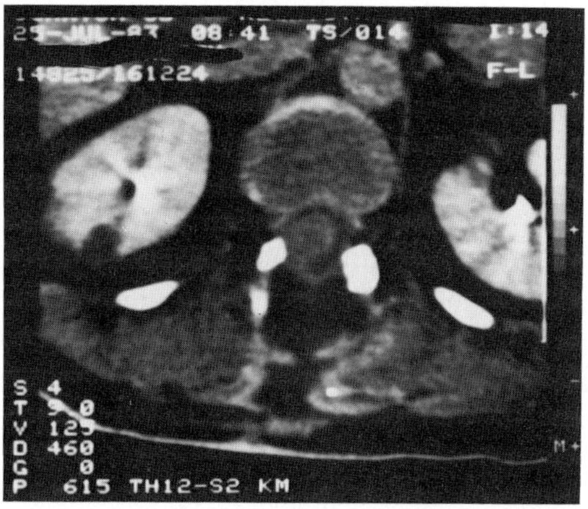

b

Fig. 3. Computer tomographic picture of a severe subfascial infection after a laminectomy. From the defect in the lamina there is an irregularly defined cavity which extends out into the subcutaneous tissue layers. *a* At the level of the vertebral body. *b* Slice at the level of the intervertebral disc. In this 42-year-old man the infection showed itself on the third day.

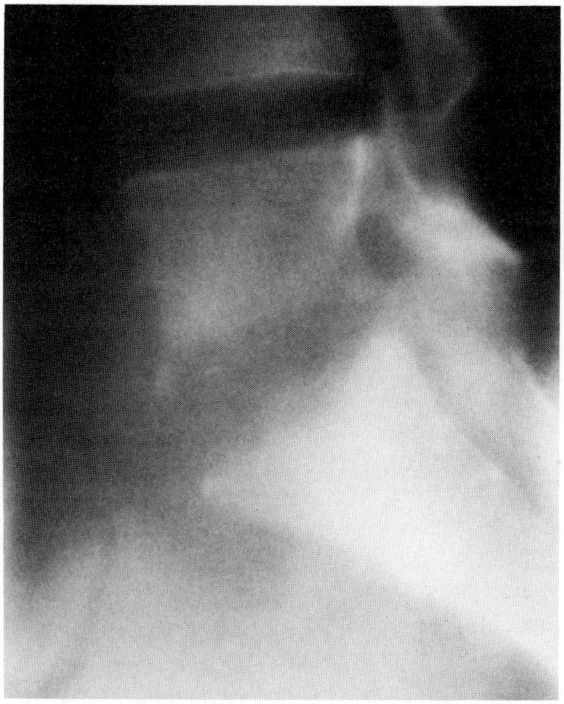

Fig. 4. Typical spondylodiscitis in the radiograph of a 39-year-old woman after an operation for a prolapsed disc at the L5/S1 level. One can see the loss of contours of the adjoining surfaces of the vertebral bodies.

In summary, it may be said that there has been no indication for perioperative prophylaxis in the typical operations in our speciality on the spinal column and the skull. The giving of antibiotics should only be considered individual cases. It is of course essential in the case of extirpation of a brain abscess in the chronic stage.

Prophylaxis in the Case of Partially Aseptic Operations and Definitely Contaminated Wounds

With contaminated wounds around the skull, urgent of course in the case of open craniocerebral injuries, we approve of prophylaxis. Here the treatment is started as soon as possible after the admission of the patient and after his examination, so that by the time of the operative procedure sufficiently high tissue levels are present. Often, bacterially contaminated foreign bodies have been carried into the wound. No prophylactic antibiotics are a substitute for a painstaking surgical revision [20]!

As regards contaminated wounds of the spinal column the same basic principles apply as in orthopedics.

We should mention here a special neurosurgical problem, namely the prophylaxis of nasal or otogenic fluid fistulas, resulting from frontobasal or lateral basal fractures [32, 46]. Here the prophylaxis should prevent the ascent of the organisms and the resultant meningitis. I regard it as absurd and dangerous to continue prophylactic treatment over a period of weeks. Should just a period of days be bridged over to the time of operation, then such treatment can perhaps be justified. We have seen meningitis not only without, but also with, prophylactic antibiotics. One must, however, be aware that this indication is not proven [26] and by the selection more dangerous and more resistant organisms probably also have their risks. Personally, I do not hold these indications as acceptable [46].

Occasionally, the opening during a craniotomy of potentially infected nasal cavities, such as the frontal sinus, cannot be avoided. Even if this often causes no trouble, one should nevertheless proceed as in the case of a partly aseptic operation, and apart from the local measures such as blocking off and covering over, undertake a prophylaxis, although possibly the time of giving the antibiotics is no longer absolutely favorable.

Specific Indications for a Prophylaxis

Here we include in the first place those patients who require the operative implantation of foreign material, with a high risk of infection [24, 41, 42].

This situation exists in the case of all shunt procedures for the treatment of various forms of hydrocephalus. Nowadays, it is self-evident that one should only use shunt systems which are sterilized by the manufacturers.

As table III shows, the infection rate is not small [21, 25]. The infection which develops during the operation, becomes clinically manifest after some days or sometimes even later. In most clinics this is just under or around 10% [14, 22], which for a primary aseptic procedure is

Table III. Inflammatory complications of shunt treatment of hydrocephalus [data from ref. 47]

	Rate %		Number of operations	Clinic
1 Infections				
Local	5.3	10.2	325	Mainz (1975–1982)
Generalized	4.9			
2 Infections	7.9		453	Hannover (1973–1981) [13]
3 Infections				
Shunt sepsis	15.2 (!)		–	Erlangen (1981) [25]
4 Infections				
(local, generalized, sepsis)	11.13		449	Göttingen

certainly too high. The inflammatory late complications such as so-called valve sepsis are likewise too common. The mode of onset is, as a rule, different from the infections which arise intra-operatively. The infection of this system in the cases of late complications results without exception from a bacteriemia with colonisation of the thrombus around the cardiac catheter. Systemic antibiotic treatment cannot eliminate the bacterial colonisation in the majority of cases, any more than the injecting of antibiotics into the shunt system. The colonisation of the shunt system and of the ensheathing thrombus, and likewise the clinical correlate of the valve sepsis can only be eliminated by the removal of the shunt. The valve system is replaced for a period of 8–10 days by a preliminary ventricular drainage, and then a new valve is implanted. In this procedure there is a very clear indication for perioperative prophylaxis [12, 13].

One should avoid all attempts at treatment by injection into the shunt system, as they practically never achieve any success. The administration of antibiotics via the CSF is in most cases of no value at all, as the infection involves the venous end of the circulation (vena cava, right auricle).

The necessity for a radical removal of the system applies equally in the case of an infected ventriculoperitoneal shunt. Here a perforation of the gut or even a bacterial invasion as a result of pressure damage to the intestinal wall can occasionally lead to abscesses or even peritonitis. Meningitis through ascending infection has frequently been described. The frequency of infection necessitating revision of the cardiac catheter stands third in the causes at 9%; on the other hand, the peritoneal catheter is in the first place with 20%. These figures from large groups of patients were published in 1978. In our clinic they are much lower at 3.2 and 12.4%, respectively. Any prophylaxis here is not particularly promising, as these are essentially late complications [28, 31, 36, 41].

The incidence of infection in freshly implanted shunt systems is one of the few indications in neurosurgery which has been checked by controlled studies [1, 19, 30]. In the present state of things I consider that perioperative prophylaxis, by the administration of a single dose, is indicated in shunt implantations. We are at present undertaking a controlled randomised study of this problem

Prophylaxis in Patients with Lowered Resistance

It is well known that immunosuppression in the field of transplantation surgery plays an important role, but less so that neurosurgical patients to no lesser degree are included among such patients. We produce, actually, a very marked immunosuppression [33] by the treatment of brain edema with high doses of dexamethasone. This should not be the occasion for prophylaxis to be demanded and carried out in all these patients. Rather, one should be much more careful with the administration of steroids, where their use is not certain or controversial, or else is attended by disadvantages, as for instance in traumatic brain edema.

A further problem is posed by those patients who are receiving cytostatic chemotherapy. At present, the most effective substances in the group of the nitrosoureas are strongly myelotoxic. The treatment is often accompanied by leucopenia and thrombocytopenia, and not uncommonly there is also anemia. It is true that these complications are, without exception, controllable; nevertheless, in the case of an urgent operation intervention in the phase of bone marrow depression there is an increased risk of infection, even in the case of strictly aseptic procedures. However, in these cases there does not appear to be any clear indication for a perioperative prophylaxis.

Practical Implementation of Perioperative Prophylaxis

It should be stressed that in the special field of neurosurgery indications indeed exist and are well substantiated, but there are very few qualitatively convincing studies [16, 34].

We are in agreement with the view of the majority of surgically orientated authors that such a prophylaxis should be started if possible 1–2 h before the operation and the administration can be continued for a maximum of up to 24 h. Giving it for several days is neither appropriate nor economical. In all cases the preparations must be given parenterally [15, 37].

The experiences of *Gruber* with a single dose perioperatively seem to us to be quite remarkable; up to the present time there have not been sufficient experiences of this type in our own speciality. Certainly, we must confess that in the meantime we have also overlooked this type of prophylaxis.

In the choice of antibiotics and their combinations, one has to bear in mind the fact that a definite change has been noted in the incidence of pathogens in wound infections. In neurosurgery, infections with a single agent predominate in about 65%. It is striking that there has been a fall in gram-negative bacteria and an increase in gram-positive cocci and the bacteroides. The increase in staphylococci is considerable.

In the first place we recommend a penicillin, where apart from penicillin G (10–20 mU/day i.v.), acylureido-penicillin piperacillin (6–12 g/day i.v.) or mezlocillin (6–15 g/day i.v.) can be considered above all. Often a so-called staphylococcus-penicillin an isoxazolyl-penicillin (oxacillin, flucloxacillin) (4–12 g/day i.v.) suffices. Combinations are possible with an aminoglucoside, among which we favor gentamycin (2–5 mg/kg/day) on account of the possibility of intrathecal administration. Tobramycin, amikacin and netilmycin offer only occasional advantages.

Instead of a penicillin, cephalosporins of the first generation, such as cefazedone or cefradine, are also still effective and from the preparations of the second generation cefotoxin (4–10 g/day), while cefotaxim or lamoctam should only be used specifically for 'problem organisms' (nosocomial infections). Meanwhile, chloramphenicol has indeed experienced a rehabilitation for the treatment of infections of the central nervous system, especially in pediatrics. However, I do not regard it as suitable for perioperative prophylaxis.

Parenteral, if possible intravenous, administration is required. There are good grounds, even in the speciality of neurosurgery, for checking the efficacy of 'single-dose prophylaxis'. Relevant studies are urgently necessary as the few studies available have not been well planned or undertaken.

Conclusions

In neurosurgery the following indications for a perioperative antibiotic prophylaxis appear to be reasonable: (1) Extirpation of a brain abscess. (2) Definitely or possibly contaminated wounds after compound injuries. (3) Implantation of foreign material with the risks of bacterial colonisation (shunt systems).

There are also some relative indications: (1) Patients with a reduced level of resistance (dexamethasone treatment, cytostatics). (2) If the paranasal sinuses are opened during a craniotomy (frontal sinus) in the context of a strictly aseptic operation.

A cerebrospinal fluid fistula does not represent an indication for prophylaxis with antibiotics.

Unfortunately, for the indications mentioned there are no sufficiently large, well-planned series, which would be capable of proving and quantifying the value of this prophylaxis.

We favor a perioperative 'single-dose prophylaxis', where the antibiotic should be given parenterally 1 h before the start of the operation, as a rule intravenously. In those cases in which a higher tissue level seems necessary the treatment can be continued for up to 12 h. Treatment for any longer period is not justifiable.

References

1 Ajir, F.; Levin, A.B.; Duff, T.A.: Effect of prophylactic methicillin on cerebrospinal fluid shunt infections in children. Neurosurgery *9:* 6–11 (1981).

2 Adam, D.: Antibiotics in neurosurgical infections including perioperative short term prophylaxis. Neurochirurgia *24:* suppl., p. 326 (1981).

3 Bergmann, B.R.: Antibiotic prophylaxis in open and closed fractures: a controlled clinical trial. Acta orthop. scand. *53:* 57–62 (1982).

4 Brand, B.; Johnson, J.T.: Prophylactic perioperative antibiotics in contaminated head and neck surgery. Trans. Pa. Acad. Ophthalmol. Otolaryngol. *35:* 51–54 (1982).

5 Brand, R.A.; Peres, H., Jr.: Antibioticos profilaticos em neurocirurgia. Arq. neuropsiquiatr. *37:* 42–47 (1979).
6 Cruse, P.: Antibiotic prophylaxis in aseptic surgery – indicated or not? Akt. Probl. clin. Orthop. *19:* 57–58 (1981).
7 Daschner, F.: Perioperative Antibiotikaprophylaxe: Eine Dosis, ein Tag oder mehrere Tage? Klinikarzt *4:* 255–256 (1983).
8 Dipiro, J.T.; Record, K.E.; Schanzenbach, K.S.; Bivins, B.A.: Antimicrobial prophylaxis in surgery. Part 2. Am. J. hosp. Pharm. *38:* 487–494 (1981).
9 Everett, E.D.; Strausbaugh, L.J.: Antimicrobial agents and the central nervous system. Neurosurgery *6:* 691–714 (1980).
10 Faden, H.: Prophylactic antibiotics in pediatric orthopedic surgery: current practices. Infect. Control *2:* 107–109 (1981).
11 Freylejer, A.; Ginesin, M.L.; Rios, J.F.: The treatment of surgical infections by deep intramuscular administration of mezlocillin. Infection *10:* 141–143 (1982).
12 Friedrich, H.; Haensel-Friedrich, G.: Perioperative chemoprophylaxis in shunting-infections. Adv. Neurosurg. *6:* 52–55 (1978).
13 Friedrich, H.; Haensel-Friedrich, G.; Potel, J.: Therapie der postoperativen Liquorraum-Infektionen; in Voth, Gutjahr, Glees, Hydrocephalus im frühen Kindesalter, pp. 303–307 (Enke, Stuttgart 1983).
14 George, R.; Leibrock, L., Epstein, M: Long-term analysis of cerebrospinal fluid shunt infections. A 25-year experience. J. Neurosurg. *51:* 804–811 (1979).
15 Gorbach, S.L.: Prophylactic antibiotics-indications in surgical patients. Scand. J. infect. Dis., suppl. pp. 134–140 (1982).
16 Guglielmo, B.J.; Hohn, D.C.; Koo, P.J.; et al.: Antibiotic prophylaxis in surgical procedures, a critical analysis of the literature. Archs Surg. *118:* 943–955 (1983).
17 Haines, S.J.: Systemic antibiotic prophylaxis in neurological surgery. Neurosurgery *6:* 355–361 (1980).
18 Haines, S.J.; Goodman, M.L.: Antibiotic prophylaxis of postoperative neurosurgical wound infections. J. Neurosurg. *56:* 103–105 (1982).
19 Haines, S.J.; Taylor, F.: Prophylactic methicillin for shunt operations: effects of incidence of shunt malfunction and infection. Child's Brain *9:* 10–22 (1982).
20 Haines, S.J.: Topical antibiotic prophylaxis in neurosurgery. Neurosurgery *11:* 250–253 (1982).
21 Hemmer, R.: Long-term results in the operative treatment of hydrocephalus in children. Adv. Neurosurg. *8:* 155–163 (1980).
22 Herter, T.; Altenburg, H.: The diagnostic value of computerized tomography in follow-up studies after CSF drainage. Adv. Neurosurg. *10:* 147–155 (1982).
23 Horwitz, N.H.; Curtin, J.A.: Prophylactic antibiotics and wound infections following laminectomy for lumbar disc herniation. J. Neurosurg. *43:* 727–731 (1975).
24 Kessel, G.; Schwarz, M.; Voth, D.: Das Ommaya-Reservoir und seine Bedeutung für die intrathekale Zytostatikatherapie. Chirurgische Aspekte und Komplikationen; in Voth, Krauseneck, Chemotherapy of Gliomas (Gruyter, Berlin, in press 1984).
25 Klinger, M.; Kunze, S., Schneider, C.: Beeinflussende Faktoren bei der Ventilsepsis; in Voth, Gutjahr, Glees, Der Hydrocephalus im frühen Kindesalter, pp. 308–312 (Enke, Stuttgart 1983).

26 Ljunggren, K.: Liquorrhea, a review of 66 cases. Acta neurochir. *51:* 173–185 (1980).
27 Luby, J.P.: Antibiotic therapy in neurosurgical infections. Clin. Neurosurg. *28:* 87–97 (1981).
28 Mahlmann, E.G.; Schwarz, M.; Voth, D.: Intestinale und pleurale Komplikationen der peritonealen Shunttherapie; in Voth, Gutjahr, Glees, Hydrocephalus im frühen Kindesalter, pp. 277–281 (Enke, Stuttgart, 1983).
29 Malis, L.I.: Prevention of neurosurgical infections by intraoperative antibiotics. Neurosurgery *5:* 339–343 (1979).
30 McCullough, D.C.; Kane, J.G.; Presper, J.H.; Wells, M.: Antibiotic prophylaxis in ventricular shunt surgery. I. Reduction of operative infection rates with methicillin. Child's Brain *7:* 182–189 (1980).
31 Meinig, G.; Kretzschmar, K.; Samii, M.; Wallenfang, T.; Hülse, R.; Schürmann, K.: Spondylodiscitis - lumbar disc removal. Adv. Neurosurg. *4:* 55–58 (1977).
32 Miles, J.P; Garretson, H.D.; Shields, C.B.; Albright, A.L.; Prophylactic antibiotics in basilar skull fracture. Neurosurgery *8:* 495–499 (1981).
33 Miller, T.E.; North, D.K.: Clinical infections, antibiotics and immunosuppression: a puzzling relationship. Am. J. Med. *71:* 334–336 (1981).
34 Poza, M.; Aleman, F.; Martinez-Lage, M.: Prophylactic treatment with antibiotics in neurological surgery. Neurochirurgia *24:* supl., p. 12 (1981).
35 Quartey, G.R.C.; Polyzoidis, K.: Intraoperative antibiotic prophylaxis in neurosurgery. A clinical study. Neurosurgery *8:* 669–671 (1981).
36 Rama, B.; Spoerri, O.: Surgical treatment and longterm results in children with hydrocephalus. Adv. Neurosurg. *8:* 227–230 (1980).
37 Savitz, M.H.; Katz, S.S.: Rationale for prophylactic antibiotics and neurosurgery. Neurosurgery *9:* 142–144 (1981).
38 Schepelmann, F.; Greiner, L.; Pia, H.W.: Complications following operation of herniated lumbal discs. Adv. Neurosurg. *4:* 52–54 (1977).
39 Simchen, E.; Shapiro, M.; Michel, J.; Sacks, T.G.: The successful use of antibiotic prophylaxis in selected high-risk surgical patients under non-trial everyday conditions. J. hosp. Infect *1:* 211–220 (1980).
40 Sollmann, H.; Böckem, F.K.; Schmidt, K.: Problems of hospitalism in neurosurgical intensive care. Adv. Neurosurg. *2:* 343–348 (1975).
41 Strahl, E.W.; Liesegang, J.; Roosen, K.: Complications following ventriculo-peritoneal shunts. Adv. Neurosurg. *6:* 6–9 (1978).
42 Tabara, Z.B.: Postoperative infection in shunts for hydrocephalus. Are prophylactic antibiotics necessary? Br.med. J. *285:* 295 (1982).
43 Urciuoli, R.; Lo Russo, G.; Zeme, S.; Lanotte, M.: Traitement antibiotique prophylactique des complications infectieuses post-opèratoires en neurochirurgie. Agressologie *24:* 237–238 (1983).
44 Voth, D.: Antibiotika in der Neurochirurgie; in Antibiotika, pp. 213–222 (Aesopusverlag, Milan 1974).
45 Voth, D.: New aspects on antibiotic therapy in neurological surgery; in Dietz, Metzel, Langmaid, Neurological surgery, pp. 326-330 (Thieme, Stuttgart 1981).
46 Voth, D.: Neurosurgery of the frontobasal CSF fistula; in Vecsei, Fractures of the Frontobasis, pp. 26–32 (Informatica, Vienna 1983).

47 Voth, D.; Gutjahr, P.; Glees, P.: Hydrocephalus im frühen Kindesalter (Enke, Stuttgart 1983).

48 Voth, D.: Perioperative prevention of infection with antibiotics in neurosurgery. Proc. 13th Int. Congr. Chemotherapy, Vienna 1983.

49 Wallenfang, T.; Reulen, H.J.; Schürmann, K.: Therapy of brain abscess. Adv. Neurosurg. *9:* 41–47 (1981).

50 Watts, J.M.; McDonald, P.J.; O'Brien, P.E.; Marshall, V.R.; Finlay-Jones, J.J.: Infection in surgery. Basic and clinical aspects, pp. 115–129 (Churchill-Livingstone, Edinburgh 1981).

Prof. Dr. D. Voth, Neurochirurgische Klinik und Poliklinik,
Johannes Gutenberg-Universität, Langenbeckstrasse 1, D-6500 Mainz (FRG)

Antibiot. Chemother., vol. 33, pp. 184–197 (Karger, Basel 1985)

Perioperative Prevention of Infection in Ophthalmic Surgery

T.M. Radda, M.M. Grasl, H.D. Gnad

Ist Department of Ophthalmology, University Hospital, Vienna, Austria

Introduction

Over the last several decades, the incidence of postoperative infection of the eye in the well-developed countries has apparently decreased from greater than 10% to acceptable levels of 0.1–0.3% [1]. The decrease in the number of cases of infectious endophthalmitis has been attributed to improved sterile operative management, including the praeoperative scrub of the surgeon's hands, the wearing of gloves, the sterilization of instruments and air, improved surgical techniques, and at least the use of pre- and postoperative antibiotics.

However, vision is still lost through ocular infections in spite of the vast number of chemotherapeutic and antibiotic substances available. A large percentage (up to 50%) of these agents administered all over the world are given to prevent infection, rather than to treat established disease. This practice led to misuse of these drugs, but on the other hand, it is not always practical to identify a bacterial or fungal infection clearly before treatment must be initiated.

The goal of perioperative antibiotic prophylaxis underlies the idea that it is essentially easier to prevent bacterial colonization rather than to decontaminate postoperative contaminated tissue which is poorly supplied with blood. However, primarily the risk of side effects of the chemotherapeutic agent has to be carefully and critically evaluated against the risk of possible infection.

Table I. Potential sources of the most common culture-positive isolates in endophthalmitis

Gram-positive	Gram-negative	Fungi
Staphylococcus aureus[1]	*Pseudomonas aeruginosa*	*Aspergillus flavus*
Staphylococcus epidermidis	*Proteus* spp.	*Fusarium* spp.
Streptococcus spp.	*Haemophilus influenzae*	*Candida*
Bacillus spp.	*Serratia marcescens*	mixed
40–60%	20–30%	10–15%

[1] Up to 80% penicillinase producing.

Indications for Perioperative Antibiotic Prophylaxis

Several factors determine the size of a critical number of bacteria in the wound at the time of closure. These include the virulence of the bacteria, the presence of devitalized or poorly vascularized tissue, the presence of a foreign body, and the status of the host defense mechanisms.

Justifications for perioperative antibiotic prophylaxis are: (1) the extent of contamination; (2) post-traumatic with penetrating trauma of the globe; (3) duration of operation; (4) functional state of the host's defense mechanism: (a) quality of humoral and cellular immunity; (b) local factors (pus, hemoglobin, anaerobic conditions, presence of a foreign body); (c) advanced age, suboptimal nutrition and poor general health; (d) genetic factors, pregnancy, disorders of the nervous system and drug allergy; (e) patients with serious neoplastic disease, severe metabolic disturbance such as diabetes mellitus; and (5) surgical procedures with statistically higher incidence of infection, extensive operative procedures, and multiple operations, particularly performed within short intervals.

Several factors are important to the effective and judicious use of antibiotics to prevent infection [2]. (a) Antimicrobial activity must be present at the wound side at the time of its closure. Therefore, it is recommended that the drug should be given immediately preoperatively and intraoperatively. (b) The antibiotic must be active against most of the contaminating microorganisms. (c) There is growing evidence that the continued use of drugs after the surgical procedure is unwarranted. Prolonged use does, however, lead to the development of a more resistant flora and of wound infections caused by antibiotic-resistant strains, and, of course, to a high risk of toxicity and unnecessary expense.

After determination, in which case a perioperative antibiotic prophylaxis is indicated, the following considerations for selection of an antibiotic agent are to be taken into account: first, which strain(s) account(s) for infection in the most common operations in eye surgery (see table I); second, which antibiotic agents cover these strains; third, factors affecting the intraocular penetration of an antibiotic agent, and fourth, starting and duration of prophylaxis (prolongation).

Incidence of Intraocular Infection

Postoperative endophthalmitis is a dreaded complication of any intraocular surgery. In cataract surgery, most reports show an impressive decline to 0.05–0.2% in the rate of bacterial postoperative infections [3, 4], which is attributed to improved sterilization technique and utilization of preoperative and periocular prophylactic antibiotics. There is a notably higher incidence of culture-positive infections in patients following intraocular lens implantation compared with routine intracapsular cataract extraction [5]. Problems related to intraocular lenses are two forms of postoperative uveitis. The more common form, a prolonged low-grade uveitis, is associated with anterior chamber reaction, lens precipitates, vitreous condensation, and cystoid macular edema. The much more severe uveitic syndrome is the postoperative sterile hypopyon, which typically appears a few days after surgery and mimics endophthalmitis [6].

A substantial tenfold decrease in the incidence of endophthalmitis after intracapsular cataract extraction has been achieved with routine intracameral injection of small quantities of gentamicin (50 μg) in eye camp cataract extraction [7]. Although most infections appear immediately following surgery, intraocular infections may be delayed for weeks or years after the operation. *Dunnington and Regan* [8] noted the danger of late-onset infection in the presence of a fistula.

After glaucoma surgery, a thin-walled bleb and hypotonous eyes are the most common contributing factors to the development of infection. The incidence of late-onset infection after Elliot's fistulizing operation for chronic glaucoma occutrred in 2–3% of the cases and is therefore nowadays obsolete [9]. Endogenous courses of postoperative complications include the surgical trauma (scleral cautery, cyclodiathermy), iris adhesions and vitreous adhesions. Contributing factors are trauma to the blebs in patients wearing contact lenses, diabetic patients or an increased bacterial fungal flora from chronic inflammation of the eye adnexes.

Endophthalmitis associated with penetrating keratoplasty is usually rare, sporadic reports have described cases in which bacteria or fungi were transferred from donor to host. Contamination of donor corneas, both from postmortem eyes or stored in McCarey-Kaufmann medium might be the source of infection.

Infection after Retinal Detachment Surgery

A mild iridocyclitis is normal and clears with topical steroids within 2 or 3 weeks. The incidence of an early extra- and intraocular infection following a scleral buckling procedure is upto 3.4% [10]. The acute postoperative bacterial infection has to be distinguished from other causes of intraocular inflammation after detachment surgery, particularly acute severe uveitis after excessive cryotherapy. The major point of differentiation between sterile uveitis and real bacterial infection is the absence of a mucopurulent discharge, an occurrence not usually until the fifth day, and a rapid resolution of the symptoms by systemic steroids. In the event of an acute scleral abscess, which is manifest by a creamy-yellow appearence to the portions of the retina overlying the buckle and a rapidly progressive exudate in the surrounding vitreous, patients require removal of the implants immediately and local and systemic antibiotic therapy for several days (e.g. gentamicin 2 × 40 mg parabulbar and 3 × 80 mg i.m. and ticarcillin 3 × 5 g i.v.). Depending on the degree of vitreous reaction, systemic steroids (50–75 mg prednisolone i.v./day during 1 week) may be beneficial.

Predisposing factors for buckle infections are the quantity of silicone material included in the operation, reoperations, with a 5 times higher incidence of infection [11], poor suturing technique and the presence of a thin sclera.

The risk of an intraocular infection increases by prolonged surgery (e.g. vitrectomy, gas-fluid exchange, subretinal drainage and lamellar scleral resection in patients with massive proliferative vitreoretinopathy particularly suffering from diabetes mellitus). *Hitchings* et al. [15] could reduce the high incidence of both extra- and intraocular infection by injecting a single dose of 40 mg gentamicin below Tenon's capsule in the quadrant surrounding the sponges at the end of operation as an antibiotic prophylaxis. Once an infection develops, the implanted material requires surgical removal, which is usually curative in cases of extraocular infection.

Infection after Vitrectomy

The reported incidence of endophthalmitis after closed vitrectomy is rare and ranges from 0.14 to 1.0% [12]. About 75% of the cases with postoperative intraocular infection are diabetic. Early ocular signs of postvitrectomy bacterial endophthalmitis are easily masked by their similarity to normal postvitrectomy reactions. The pain that signals intraocular infection is easily mistaken for the usual postoperative ocular discomfort and is frequently overlooked. Hypopyon seems to develop more frequently and more rapidly in aphakic than in phakic eyes. An increased inflammation may result not only from the vitreous instrumentation itself, but also from the increased time, in the utilization of air, gas and intraocular solutions.

As soon as endophthalmitis seems a possibility, antimicrobial prophylaxis, pre- and intraoperatively, prompt diagnostic vitreous aspiration, followed by the use of intravitreal and systemic broad-spectrum antibiotics, should be done.

Post-Traumatic Endophthalmitis

The indicence of infectious endophthalmitis following penetrating trauma varies considerably. In a retrospective series of 87 consecutive cases of penetrating trauma, *Forster* [4] found only 2 (2.4%) with cultured proved endophthalmitis *(Staphylococcus epidermidis, Enterobacter agglomerans).* 77 of 82 cases were treated prophylactically with cephalothin intravenously as well as with parabulbar gentamicin and topical antibiotics. *Brinton* et al. [13] reported that 10.7% of patients

Table II. Potential sources of infection during eye surgery [from *Forster*, 5]

Ambient air
Respiratory origin
Surface origin (e.g. skin, clothing)
Air-conditioning system
Solutions and medications
Saline for Irrigation and other purposes
Collyria
Ointments
Instrument desinfectants
Skin antiseptics
Tissues
Skin of hands
Skin of operative field
Lid margins and lashes
Conjunctival sac
Lacrimal sac
Nasal mucosa
Corneal grafts (fresh or medium cultured)
Vitreous implants (e.g. silicone oil, healon)
Objects and materials
Optical instruments
Surgical instruments
Tonometers
Magnets
Hypodermic needles, blood lancets
Cotton balls, swabs, drapes, dressings masks and gowns
Rubber gloves, bulbs, droppers
Glass syringes, bottles, irrigation tips
Plastic tubing, sheeting, retractors
Orbital implantats
Intraocular lenses
Sutures

with intraocular foreign bodies and 5.2% without an intraocular foreign body had developed endophthalmitis. It is surprising that there are not more cases of endophthalmitis after penetrating trauma. It is suggested that high-velocity metal fragments sterilize themselves when generated from the impact. If a metal object or other foreign material penetrates the globe, one might consider a bacterial infection. Wood or other vegetable matter may harbour fungi [14]. Pain seems to be an important symptom in the diagnosis of most bacterial infections. A delay-

Table III. Medical treatment and recommended antibiotic combinations[1] for prophylaxis of endophthalmitis after penetrating trauma

Systemic[2]	Topical	Subconjunctival/parabulbar	Intravitreal/ intracameral	Oral[3]
Gentamicin, 80 mg every 8 h i.m.	gentamicin, 3%	gentamicin, 40 mg once or twice a day	gentamicin, 0.1 mg	prednisolone 100–200 mg
or	or	or	cefazolin, 2.5 mg	
Amikacin, 500 mg twice a day	amikacin, 5%	amikacin, 25–50 mg/day		
		with		
Cefazolin, 1.5 g		cefazolin, 100 mg/day		
or		or		
Cefotaxim, 2 g every 6 h		cefotaxim, 100 mg/day		
		and		
		clindamycin, 34 mg/day (if there is an intraocular foreign body)		

[1] The choice of antibiotics is determined by the in vitro sensitivity of the organism.
[2] For an averaged-sized adult with normal renal function.
[3] 1 day after beginning antibiotics.

ed onset of inflammation, with or without pain, appears to be more indicative of anaerobes, low-virulence organisms, and fungi.

Prognostic factors include the virulence of the organisms, the duration of time between onset of endophthalmitis and starting prompt and aggressive treatment, the type and severity of injury, with or without retinal break or detachment, and the type of treatment given [14].

A list of the very recently recommended antibiotic combinations for prophylaxis of posttraumatic endophthalmitis is given in table III. The maximum nontoxic dose of antibiotic and antifungal agents for vitrectomy infusion fluid for endophthalmitis is listed in table IV.

Etiology-Pathogenesis

The etiologic agents in acute postoperative, late-onset postoperative, traumatic or metastatic endophthalmitis include bacteria, fungi and noninfectious factors. Whether the intraocular inflammation is in-

Table IV. Maximum nontoxic dose of antibiotic and antifungal agents for vitrectomy infusion fluid for endophthalmitis [from *Peyman* et al., 7]

	Nontoxic dose, μg/ml
Single	
Chloramphenicol	10
Clindamycin	9
Amikacin	10
Tobramycin	10
Gentamicin	8
Methicillin	20
Lincomycin	10
Oxacillin	10
Penicillin G	10
Amphothericin B	75[1]
Combination	
1 Gentamicin	8
Oxacillin	10
2 Clindamycin	9
Gentamicin	8
3 Methicillin	20
Gentamicin	8

[1] Recommended dose is 10 μg/ml.

fectious or sterile in origin needs exact determination. Only culture-positive isolates from the anterior chamber, the vitreous, or open dehiscent wounds indicate a causative etiology. Cultures obtained from conjunctivae, wound area or smears do not prove a bacterial or fungal etiology. The potential sources of infection during eye surgery are summarized in table II.

Types of Infection

Bacterial. In table I the most common culture-positive isolates causing endophthalmitis are summarized. Of the gram-positive organisms, penicillinase-producing *Staphylococcus aureus* is the most frequent agent responsible for endophthalmitis. Thus, initial therapy and prophylaxis should be directed at penicillinase-producing organisms. Antibiotics effective against these organisms include the penicillinase-resistant penicillins (methicillin, oxacillin), the cephalosporins, vancomycin, lincomycin, clindamycin, tetracyclins, chloramphenicol and recently fosfomycin, which seems to penetrate the aqueous and vitreous to a much greater level than do the penicillins, aminoglycosides or cephalosporins. Agents of lesser pathogenicity, such as *S. epidermidis*, may produce a more delayed, indolent inflammatory reaction, whereas *Pseudomonas aeruginosa* and *S. aureus* present a fulminating course and progress rapidly.

Gram-negative infections of the eye are mainly due to *P. aeruginosa* or *Proteus.* Usually, Pseudomonas is sensitive to the aminoglycosides gentamicin, tobramycin, amikacin and netilmicin and to a lesser extent carbenicillin and ticarcillin. With increasing specific diagnosis, additional etiologic agents are being described. With the frequent use of antibiotics and steroids, especially in the postoperative period, organisms previously considered nonvirulent may in fact be pathogenic to the eye. A metastatic *Serratia marcescens* endophthalmitis occurred in a man with chronic lymphatic leukemia after prostatectomy and diabetes mellitus type II for 3 years [16]. There are also increasing reports of isolates which indicate the potential for common, ubiquitous organisms to be infectious agents in endophthalmitis. *Forster* [4] associated 3 cases of *Haemophilus influenzae* infection in filtering blebs after glaucoma surgery and two bacillus species associated with trauma.

In conclusion, any organism is probably capable of producing infection if suitably inoculated into a susceptible eye by trauma, postoperative or metastatic, in immunoincompetent patients. Delayed infections may be due to poor personal hygiene, persistent filtering cicatrices, or the vitreous wick syndrome, a late complication following cataract extraction. Blood, fibrin, or lens material provide nutrients for bacterial contamination and multiplication.

Fungal. A fungal etiology for postinjury or postsurgery infection is quite rare, even if the fungus is in oculated immediately during intraocular surgery, the onset of clinical symptoms may be delayed for months. A higher incidence of metastatic fungal endophthalmitis is reported from patients receiving immunosuppressive agents, systemic antibiotics or corticosteroids for a long period of time.

Sterile. A sterile, postoperative iridocyclitis and vitreous inflammation presents the most difficult differential diagnostic problem. A sterile non-infectious etiology of postoperative and postinjury inflammation might be due to retained lenticular material, excessive vitreous manipulation, wound incarceration of lenticular, iris or vitreous material, foreign material, such as talc, starch or chemicals, or residual polishing compounds of intraocular lens implants. Foreign bodies and deposition of environmental material may produce toxic, noninfectious inflammation following trauma. With the increase in extracapsular cataract surgery, phacoemulsification and implantation of anterior or posterior chamber lenses, the sterile type of postoperative inflammation becomes more common.

Clinical Manifestation

Clinical symptoms in bacterial endophthalmitis include a sudden onset of increasing pain, hyperemia, lidedema, conjunctival chemosis, clouding of the aqueous and the vitreous, and secondary glaucoma. Though pain is a common feature of bacterial endophthalmis, it is often absent in patients with endophthalmitis occurring months or years after filtering surgery, fistulizing wounds or with unrecognized vitreous wick syndrome. Hypopyon, blurred vision, lacrimation and fever are other characteristic manifestations of endophthalmitis. In contrast to the rapid development of bacterial endophthalmitis, fungal infection shows only slow depression of visual function and a gradual onset, transient hypopyon and cotton balls on the vitreous face and iris.

An apparently sterile uveitis, postoperative or post-traumatic, might be the precursor of a veritable severe intraocular infection. Changing of the hazy aqueous or vitreous to yellow and formation of a mucopurulent discharge in the following postoperative days prove the development of endophthalmitis. To separate sterile endophthalmitis from cases suspect of been infectious, a careful clinical examination and experience are necessary. However, if any infection is suspected, diagnostic cultures are necessary, and therapy should be started immediately.

Prophylaxis of Postoperative Intraocular Infection

Antibiotic agents should be bactericidal for the infecting organism, should have no significant toxicity, and adequate levels of the antibiotic should be achieved in the various compartments and tissues of the eye [17].

Local Management

(1) If conjunctivitis, chalazia, blepharitis, acne or dacryocystitis is present, it should be treated and cleared before surgery. (2) Chemical preparation of the eye reduces a number of infecting organism on lid margin and lashes significantly [18]. (3) Since the normal flora includes the wide range of bacteria on the patient's lid and conjunctiva, both pathogenic and 'nonpathogenic', every eye should be considered as potentially contamined and should be pretreated with antibiotics to reduce or eliminate contaminants. The more popular combined antibiotic preparations are those combining neomycin, polymyxin B and bacitracin in solution form. *Allen and Mangiaracine* [3] presented convincing evidence to support the use of preoperative antibiotics topically before surgery. (4) Diabetics and patients with skin diseases should be specially questioned and examined regarding infections. (5) A routine use of preoperative cultures has been widely discussed. However, the routine use of preoperative cultures is probably not practical or beneficial, since *S. epidermidis* is usually found in 50–70% and *S. aureus* in approximately 30% of normal eyes. The knowledge of preoperative cultures gives the surgeon a false sense of security, since there are no data to relate preoperative cultures to the specific etiologic agent in postoperative endophthalmitis [4].

Preoperative Management

A short time use (1–3 days pre- and postoperatively) of a broad-spectrum antibacterial agent e.g. a prophylactic systemic antibiotic such as gentamicin, seems rational in treating enteric gram-negative rods, *P. aeruginosa,* and penicillinase-producing *Staphylococcus* species. The increasing of resistant strains of staphylococcus may be a problem if gentamicin is used for a long-term management. In infections caused by gram-negative rods, gentamicin offers a broader spectrum of activity than polymixin B and in addition is active against staphylococci. A currently popular choice is gentamicin, 40 mg in 1 ml of saline solution for subconjunctival injection.

Although prophylactic subconjunctival antibiotics have traditionally been given at the end of cataract surgery, a more rational time of injection is just before surgery. This timing permits antibiotic action during the dangerous period when the eye is open and makes the antibiotic immediately available for penetration into the eye as the blood-aqueous barrier is broken down by the incision.

Although gentamicin has been proved to be effective in many ocular inflammations, some strains of gram-negative organisms have demonstrated the ability to synthesize antibiotic-inactivating enzymes. Amikacin and netilicin are newer potent aminoglycoside antibiotics efficient against many gentamicin-resistant strains. Amikacin has a broad-spectrum bactericidal activity against *S. aureus, P. aeruginosa, Proteus* spp., *Escherichia coli, Klebsiella* and *Enterobacter* spp. and *Serratia marcescens* [19]. After intramuscular injection of 15 mg/kg/day of amikacin, the concentration reaches levels in human primary aqueous humor equivalent or much higher (up to 5 times) than the medium minimum inhibitory concentration against most of the pathogens causing bacterial endophthalmitis. For preoperative prophylaxis, therapeutic levels can be reached in the aqueous humor for about 6 h after intramuscular application of 15 mg/kg amikacin. *Peyman* et al. [14] concluded that intravitreal administration of amikacin is the most effective route for prophylaxies and treatment of postoperative infections and they demonstrated that intravitreal injection of 250 mg amikacin produced no histological, ophthalmic or electroretinographic evidence of toxicity in the rabbit eye. Netilmicin, particularly in combination with β-lactamantibiotics, reaches levels equivalent to a minimum inhibitory concentration of common organisms.

Recently, there has also been the possibility of intravitreal aminoglycoside application in the course of a vitrectomy [20]. During this process the vitreous is aspirated and is replaced by diluted antibiotic solutions. Combined therapeutic vitrectomy and intraocular antibiotics offer a significant break through in the management of suspected infectious endophthalmitis.

If a fungal etiology is evident, vitrectomy for both diagnostic and therapeutic purposes is performed initially with intraocular injection of both gentamicin and amphothericin B (0.05–0.01 mg). The use of systemic amphothericin B therapy is a little rational, since the intraocular penetration of this agent is poor and due to its relative systemic toxicity. Subconjunctival injections of amphothericin B at a dosage of 0.5–1.0 mg penetrate sufficiently into the anterior and posterior segment of eye.

Comment

The use of a broad-spectrum, prophylactic antibiotic agent such as gentamicin, given via the subconjunctival route, seems rational. Topical and systemic use of prophylactic antibiotics in high-risk patients or after intraocular trauma may also reduce the incidence of infection. *Leopold and Apt* [21] concluded that 'if antibiotic or chemotherapeutic agents are to be used prophylactically, they must be used as an adjunct to and not a substitute for an aseptic surgical technique.

With regard to ocular penetration, more information of the various antibiotics available is required for proper selection of the appropriate antibiotic for prevention intraocular infection.

References

1 Allen, H.F.: Bacterial endophthalmitis after cataract extraction; in Bellows, Cataract and anomalities of the lens, pp. 421–428 (Grune & Stratton, New York 1975).

2 Sandusky, W.R.: Postoperative infections and antimicrobial prophylaxis for surgical infection; in Mandell, Douglas, Bennet. Principles and practice of infectious diseases, pp. 2248–2256 (Wiley, New York 1979).

3 Allen, H.F.; Mangiaracine, A.B.: Bacterial endophthalmitis after cataract extraction. II. Incidence in 36.000 consecutive operations with special reference to preoperative topical antibiotics. Archs Ophthal. *91:* 3–7 (1974).

4 Forster, R.K.: Endophthalmitis; in Duane, Clinical ophthalmology, vol. 4, pp. 1–20 (Harper & Row, New York 1981).

5 Forster, R.K.; Abbott, R.L.; Gelender, H.: Management of infectious endophthalmitis. Ophthalmology *87:* 313–319 (1980).

6 Meltzer, D.W.: Sterile hypopyon following intraocular lens surgery. Archs. Ophthal. *98:* 100–104 (1980).

7 Peyman, G.A.; Sathor, M.L.; May, D.R.: Intraocular gentamycin as intraoperative prophylaxis in south India eye camps. Br. J. Ophthal. *61:* 260–262 (1977).

8 Dunnington, J.H.; Regan, E.F.: Late fistulization of operative wounds. Diagnosis and treatment. Archs Ophthal. *43:* 407–412 (1950).

9 Havener, W.H.: Ocular pharmacology, pp. 114–185 (Mosby, St. Louis 1978).

10 Kreissig, I.; Lincoff, H.: A comparative study of sponge infections. Mod. Probl. Ophthal., vol. 20, pp. 154–156 (Karger, Basel 1979).

11 Hahn, Y.S.; Lincoff, A.; Lincoff, H.; Kreissig, I.: Infection after sponge implantation for scleral buckling. Am. J. Ophthal. *87:* 180–185 (1979).

12 Ho, P.C.; Tolentino, F.I.: Bacterial endophthalmitis after closed vitrectomy. Archs Ophthal. *102:* 207–210 (1984).

13 Brinton, G.S.; Topping, T.M.; Hyndink, R.A.; Aaberg, T.M.; Reeser, F.H.; Abrams, G.W.: Posttraumatic endophthalmitis. Archs Opththal. *102:* 547–549 (1984).

14 Peyman, G.A.; Coroll, C.P., Raichand, M.: Prevention and management of traumatic endophthalmitis. Ophthalmology *87:* 320–324 (1980).
15 Hitchings, R.A.; Levy, I.S.; Chignell, A.H.: Acute infection after retinal detachment surgery. Br. J. Ophthal. *58:* 588–590 (1974).
16 Radda, T.M.: Metastatic serratia marcescens endophthalmitis. Ophthalmologica, Basel *185:* 65–68 (1982).
17 Borza, M.: Factors affecting the intraocular penetration of antibiotics. Scand. J. infect. Dis., suppl. 14, pp. 151–159 (1978).
18 Isenberg, S.; Apt, L.: Chemical preparation of the eye in ophthalmic surgery. Archs Ophthal. *101:* 761–765 (1983).
19 Radda, T.M.; Gnad, H.D.: Amikacin levels in human aqueous humor. Arzneimittelforsch. *33:* 1607–1608 (1983).
20 Cobo, L.M.; Forster, R.K.: The clearance of intravitreal gentamicin. Am. J. Ophthal. *92:* 59–62 (1981).
21 Leopold, I.H.; Apt, L.: Postoperative intraocular infections. Am. J. Ophthal. *50:* 1225–1247 (1960).

Dr. T.M. Radda, Ist Department of Ophthalmology, Spitalgasse 2,
A-1090 Vienna (Austria)

Subject Index